Health, Technology and Society

Series Editors
Rebecca Lynch
Wellcome Centre for Cultures and Environments
of Health
University of Exeter
Exeter, UK

Martyn Pickersgill
Usher Institute
University of Edinburgh
Edinburgh, UK

Medicine, health care, and the wider social meaning and management of health are undergoing major changes. In part this reflects developments in science and technology, which enable new forms of diagnosis, treatment and delivery of health care. It also reflects changes in the locus of care and the social management of health. Locating technical developments in wider socio-economic and political processes, each book in the series discusses and critiques recent developments in health technologies in specific areas, drawing on a range of analyses provided by the social sciences. Some have a more theoretical focus, some a more applied focus but all draw on recent research by the authors. The series also looks toward the medium term in anticipating the likely configurations of health in advanced industrial society and does so comparatively, through exploring the globalization and internationalization of health.

Claudia Egher

Digital Healthcare and Expertise

Mental Health and New Knowledge Practices

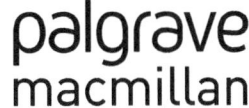

Claudia Egher
Department of Health, Ethics and Society
Maastricht University
Maastricht, The Netherlands

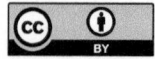

ISSN 2946-3386   ISSN 2946-3378   (electronic)
Health, Technology and Society
ISBN 978-981-16-9177-5   ISBN 978-981-16-9178-2   (eBook)
https://doi.org/10.1007/978-981-16-9178-2

This Palgrave Macmillan imprint is published by the registered company Springer Nature Singapore Pte Ltd.
The registered company address is: 152 Beach Road, #21-01/04 Gateway East, Singapore 189721, Singapore

To Véronique

Series Editors' Preface

Medicine, healthcare, and the wider social meanings and management of health are continually in the process of change. While the "birth of the clinic" heralded the process through which health and illness became increasingly subject to the surveillance of medicine, for example, surveillance has become more complex, sophisticated, and targeted—as seen in the search for "precision medicine" and now "precision public health." Both surveillance and health itself emerge as more provisional, uncertain, and risk-laden as a consequence, and we might also ask what now constitutes "the clinic," how meaningful a concept of a clinic ultimately is, and where else might we now find (or not find) healthcare spaces and interventions.

Ongoing developments in science and technology are helping to enable and propel new forms of diagnosis, treatment, and the delivery of healthcare. In many contexts, these innovations both reflect and further contribute to changes in the locus of care and burden of responsibility for health. Genetics, informatics, and imaging—to name but a few—are redefining collective and individual understandings of the body, health, and disease. At the same time, long-established and even ostensibly mundane technologies and techniques can generate ripples in local discourse and practices as ideas about the nature and focus of healthcare shift in response to global debates about, for instance, One Health and Planetary Health.

The very technologies that (re)define health are also the means through which the individualization of healthcare can occur—through, for instance, digital health, diagnostic tests, and the commodification of restorative tissue. This individualization of health is both culturally derived and state-sponsored, as exemplified by the promotion of "self-care." These shifts are simultaneously welcomed and contested by professionals, patients, and the wider public. Hence they at once signal and instantiate wider societal ambivalences and divisions.

This series explores these processes within and beyond the conventional domain of "the clinic," and asks whether they amount to a qualitative shift in the social ordering and value of medicine and health. Locating technical use and developments in wider socioeconomic and political processes, each book discusses and critiques the dynamics between health, technology, and society through a variety of specific cases and draws on a range of analyses provided by the social sciences.

The series has already published more than 20 books that have explored many of these issues, drawing on novel, critical, and deeply informed research undertaken by their authors. In doing so, the books have shown how the boundaries between the three core dimensions that underpin the whole series—health, technology, and society—are changing in fundamental ways.

In *Digital Healthcare and Expertise*, Claudia Egher focuses on an area that has attracted much promise, hope, and investment—but which nevertheless remains less well studied than might be expected within the social studies of medicine: digital mental health. This exciting monograph considers compelling questions around the construction and mediation of experiences framed often in psychiatry and beyond as "bipolar disorder" within digital spaces, with particular analytic attention to the performance and negotiation of expertise. It provides a bold analysis of the reconfiguring of (the relations between) forms of online (and offline) epistemic practices, performances of and claims to knowledge and expertise, and understandings and experiences of the self. Through *Digital Healthcare and Expertise*, Egher illustrates the complexities inherent to shifting understandings and deployments of expertise relating to bipolar disorder within online platforms, and presents a novel interpellation of science and technology studies, medical sociology, and media studies that will be vital to future analyses of health, technology, and society.

London, UK   Rebecca Lynch
Edinburgh, UK   Martyn Pickersgill

Acknowledgments

Working on this book has been an incredible adventure, and I am deeply grateful for all the help and support I have received along the way from colleagues, family, and friends, from the first stages of my doctoral research upon which this work is based to the close readings of its penultimate draft.

Having immersed myself in the experiences of people diagnosed with bipolar disorder for many years now, I have acquired a rich understanding of the challenges involved in the management of this condition. Without wanting to be presumptuous, I would therefore like to first and foremost express my gratitude to the many people diagnosed with bipolar disorder, who have written about their states, experiments, joys, and difficulties on the digital platforms I studied. In the absence of such endeavors, this book would literally not have been possible. I do hope that it does justice to their tremendous efforts and valuable insights.

I would particularly like to thank Natasha Tracy and Julie A. Fast, who kindly allowed me to interview them and use materials from their digital platforms. I can still vividly remember how impressed I was during the first year of my PhD, when I discovered their blogs and became aware of the numerous and varied contributions they were making across different media. I continue to be impressed by their work, and I would like to express my appreciation for their dedication and considerable efforts to help improve the lives of other people diagnosed with bipolar disorder.

I would also like to thank the representatives of La Haute Autorité de Santé in France, who gave me permission to reproduce materials from their website in this book.

Two chapters of *Digital Healthcare and Expertise* are the result of previously published articles that were substantially altered here. An earlier version of Chap. 4 was published in 2019 under the title "Bipolar Patients and Creative Online Practices: Sharing Experiences of Controversial Treatments" in *Health* 23(4): 458–477. A first version of Chap. 5 was published in 2020 as "Online Expert Mediators: The Rise of a New 'Bipolar' Stakeholder or Going Beyond Interactional Expertise in the Blogosphere" in *Science and Technology Studies* 33 (2): 1–22. Both articles greatly benefitted from the anonymous reviewers and from the editors at each journal, to whom I am grateful.

I owe many words of thanks to Joshua Pitt and Marion Duval, the editors I worked with on this book, as well as to the series editors, Martyn Pickersgill and Rebecca Lynch. I am also very grateful to Rubina Infanta Rani, for her patience, help, and support throughout this process. This book benefitted tremendously from the very constructive feedback and suggestions the anonymous reviewers provided on the book proposal and on the subsequent draft. My heartfelt thanks to them!

My hope is that this book will find its way and will be of relevance to medical professionals, people diagnosed with mental health conditions, policy makers, and any other stakeholder groups involved or interested in the provision of mental healthcare. I am therefore particularly grateful for the open-access publication grant provided by the Netherlands Organization for Scientific Research (NWO) and for the financial support obtained from the Maastricht University Library. I would like to thank Sally Wyatt for all the help she provided me with throughout this process. I am also very grateful to Olga Zvonareva, Bart Penders, and Klasien Horstman for their support.

The core ideas of this book were developed while I was a PhD candidate at the Faculty of Arts and Social Sciences at Maastricht University. I owe a tremendous debt of gratitude to Sally Wyatt and Tamar Sharon for their guidance, advice, unwavering support, and multiple close readings of drafts. They have been phenomenal PhD supervisors and they have inspired me ever since! The tenacity and motivation required to finish this book during the challenging times of the pandemic have been to a large extent stimulated by them. I consider myself very lucky for having made my first steps into STS under the close guidance of Wiebe Bijker, and I am deeply grateful for his help and for everything that I have learned from him. Thanks are also due to Ruud Hendriks, who inspired my first sociological forays into mental health. The shortening and sharpening of this book benefitted from the constructive feedback provided by Tsjalling Swierstra, to whom I am very grateful. I was also inspired and invigorated by the presentations and talks I have had over the years with members of the Maastricht University Science, Technology and Society Studies (MUSTS) group, of the Centre for Ethics and Politics of Emerging Technologies (EPET), and of the Netherlands Graduate Research School of Science, Technology, and Modern Culture (WTMC).

This book has also benefitted from the close reading and friendly feedback provided by very kind and generous friends. Hortense, Valentina, Lisa, Simone, and Thomas, thank you so much for all your help!

Finally, I want to express my deep love and gratitude to my family and friends, to those who have supported me through some pretty hard times and with whom I have shared countless joyful and amazing moments. Thank you for constantly reminding me that there is a life out there, while also being understanding and accepting of my need to work. Mamă și tată, vă mulțumesc pentru ajutor și susținere! Many thanks also to Lucia and Christian for the wonderfully relaxing moments spent together! One of my deep personal regrets is that Pa and my aunt Veronica are no longer with us to witness this moment. Charlie, I am extremely grateful that I could rely on your help and support throughout all the years that I worked on this book and the study preceding it. Krijn and Raquel, thank you so much for your friendship and for your willingness to read drafts, double-check references, and help with the editing and any other issue pertaining to my work for so many years now. Lori, thank you for your friendship, for your patience, and for the constant and often last-minute (sorry about that!) efforts to make my graphs and tables look better! Andreea, Oana, PJ, Nico, Julia, Luat, Bart, Laura, Bogdan, Andrei, Simona, Dina, Kosmas, Marith, Willemine, Dara, and Ricky, thank you so much for your friendship! Much love and gratitude to Hortense—it is no exaggeration to say that this book would not have been finalized, had it not been for your continuous help, encouragement, and support! I am so grateful that you're my friend! Véronique, thank you for all the drawings and jottings you left on so many of my drafts, and I'm sorry that they didn't make it into the actual manuscript. This book is for you—in the hope that one day you will understand why mummy played less often with you than you would have wanted. You are my great love!

About This Book

This book explores how expertise about bipolar disorder is performed on American and French digital platforms by combining insights from STS, medical sociology, and media studies. It addresses topical questions, including the following: How do different stakeholders engage with online technologies to perform expertise about bipolar disorder? How does the use of the Internet for processes of knowledge evaluation and production allow people diagnosed with bipolar disorder to re-position themselves in relation to medical professionals? How do cultural markers shape the online performance of expertise about bipolar disorder? And what individualizing or collectivity-generating effects does the Internet have in relation to the performance of expertise? The book thus constitutes a critical and nuanced intervention into dominant discourses which approach the Internet either as a quick technological fix or as a postmodern version of Pandora's box, sowing distrust among people and threatening unified conceptualizations and organized forms of knowledge.

Praise for *Digital Healthcare and Expertise*

"The digital era sits on an unsteady amalgam of hype and doom scenarios concerning the emancipating power of the Internet and the democratization of expertise. Claudia Egher succeeds in astutely navigating these sweeping claims to produce a more nuanced and complex picture of technologically mediated knowledge production. Her relentless search for the how, who, and where of the enactment of expertise on bipolar disorder online takes the reader on a journey that shuttles between vast theoretical literatures on expertise and the power of technology and culture to shaping it, and its actual performance. In the process, she gives voice to the new experts of bipolar disorder, where user agency is reconciled with choice architecture and solidarity persists, as a latent and stubborn dimension of individualization and personalization."

—Tamar Sharon, *Professor of Philosophy, Digitalization and Society, Radboud University Nijmegen*

"Adopting a science and technology studies approach, this intriguing book shows how expertise has different meanings to the diverse actors who are part of defining and managing bipolar disorder. As Egher's analysis demonstrates, material practices and standpoints combine to enact expertise in specific contexts. This book will be of interest to anyone who wants to know more about how expertise is multiple, dynamic, and complex."

—Deborah Lupton, *SHARP Professor in the Centre for Social Research in Health and Social Policy Research Centre, UNSW Sydney*

"This book offers a novel approach to expertise as a practical and collective achievement. With its sharp and effective focus on mental health and digital communities, it produces wide-ranging and generally applicable conclusions about expertise and the Internet's potential to democratize knowledge. The lucid description of exchanges on digital platforms on bipolar disorder makes this book a must-read for mental health professionals, STS researchers, and public health policy makers alike."

—Wiebe E. Bijker, *Professor of Technology & Society, Norwegian University of Science and Technology*

Contents

Contents

List of Acronyms and Abbreviations

AA	Alcoholics Anonymous
AI	Artificial intelligence
AIDS	Acquired immunodeficiency syndrome
APSA	L'Association des Psychotiques Stabilisés Autonomes
BPS	British Psychological Society
CESE	Conseil Économique Social et Environnemental
CNSA	Caisse Nationale de Solidarité pour l'Autonomie
DSM-5	Diagnostic and Statistical Manual of Mental Disorders, 5th edition
EBM	Evidence-based medicine
ECT	Electroconvulsive therapy
E-FOIA	Electronic Freedom of Information Act
EIT	Electronic and information technology
EMDR	Eye movement desensitization and reprocessing
EMI	Ecological momentary intervention
ERCIC	Ethical Review Committee of Inter City Faculties, Maastricht University
GDP	Gross domestic product
GDPR	General Data Protection Regulation
GEM	Groupes d'Entraide Mutuelle
GIA	Groupe d'Information Asile
GP	General practitioner
GPS	Global Positioning System

HAS   La Haute Autorité de Santé
HONcode   The Health on the Net Foundation Code of Conduct
ICD-10   The International Classification of Disease and Health Related
            Problems, 10th edition
ICT   Information and Communication Technology 9
IE   Interactional expertise
ISO   International Organization for Standardization
KTRO   Radio station licensed to transmit in Portland
LFB   Le Forum des Bipotes
NAC   N-acetylcysteine
NIMH   National Institute of Mental Health
PDF   Portable Document Format
PXE   Pseudoxanthoma elasticum
OECD   Organisation for Economic Co-operation and Development
RGAA3   Référentiel Géneral d'Accessibilité pour les Administrations
SAD   Seasonal affective disorder
STS   Science and technology studies
SEE   Studies of Expertise and Experience
UK   The United Kingdom of Great Britain and Northern Ireland
US   The United States of America
VNS   Vagus nerve stimulation
WAI   Web Accessibility Initiation
WCAG   Web Content Accessibility Guidelines
WHO   World Health Organization
W3C   World Wide Web Consortium

List of Figures

1

Studying Expertise Online

I have this med down to a science. (…) You also cannot drink any water after taking it until you wake up. You can take one swig of water here or there but I try not to. One thing that has worked for me is not eating or drinking anything from 9:30 until 12:30. This is a trial and error drug and I have schooled my doctor on what works. (*Watson*, March 9, 2015, quote slightly adapted to ensure anonymity)

As the online excerpt above suggests, the Internet has facilitated the "participatory turn" (Prainsack, 2011) in healthcare, with a plethora of online platforms and mobile health applications claimed to disrupt the traditional distribution of knowledge and power between medical professionals and people diagnosed (Dedding et al., 2011; Eysenbach et al., 2004). Yet, the term "participation" has turned out to be rather vague (Nielsen & Langstrup, 2018; Wyatt et al., 2013), and it is not clear how active such involvement with one's health is or should be, nor whether participation reaches as far as allowing people diagnosed to contribute to the production of knowledge, and what such contributions consist of. At the same time, by affording the wider circulation of scientific controversies, the Internet has contributed to a growing public awareness about the disagreements that often exist among experts and about the conditions of

© The Author(s) 2023
C. Egher, *Digital Healthcare and Expertise*, Health, Technology and Society,
https://doi.org/10.1007/978-981-16-9178-2_1

uncertainty under which they make recommendations and decisions. The Internet may have thus served both to weaken the cognitive authority of "traditional" experts and to draw attention to the fact that people lacking official accreditations can also possess substantial knowledge and experience in certain domains.

These developments are linked to the rather paradoxical position that expertise has nowadays come to occupy in Western societies. One may argue that at no other time in history has expertise been so prevalent, as it has expanded and now covers areas for which no specific and substantial knowledge was previously thought necessary, ranging from child-rearing and health to interior design, lifestyle choices, and personal savings. Yet, while this suggests that expertise has become ubiquitous as well as highly valued, the identity of experts, of those who can rightfully provide authoritative answers and solutions to complex, "wicked" problems has been challenged. As a consequence, instead of something stable and well-bounded, expertise has come to mean different things to different people: it is acquired and manifested in myriad ways across different locales, it fulfills different functions, and it is importantly shaped by social, cultural, and economic factors. This raises important questions about the identity and position of those who can acquire expertise and about the ways in which they perform it, that is, about the practices, tools, and standards through which expertise is articulated.

These elements are at the core of this book, as it asks, how is expertise about bipolar disorder performed on American and French online platforms? In so doing, it focuses on how different stakeholders engage with online technologies to perform expertise about bipolar disorder and how such activities allow them to re-position themselves in relation to medical professionals. The book further investigates the individualizing or collectivity-generating effects that the Internet has in relation to the online performance of expertise about bipolar disorder, given that it is still uncertain how it shapes such performances at the level of individuals or groups, and whether it helps give rise to new configurations. By focusing on the performance of expertise about bipolar disorder on French and American digital platforms, it also considers how cultural factors shape epistemic practices. In addressing these issues, this book contributes to the fields of science and technology studies (STS), medical sociology, and media studies. A brief overview of the public and theoretical debates that have informed these particular questions and information about how they are addressed in the chapters of this book are presented below.

The processes through which one can develop expertise are domain-specific, as they involve the acquisition of particular types of knowledge and the internalization of relevant practices, norms, and values. This book focuses on mental health, where the developments sketched above have had a profound impact, and where expertise has had a particularly convoluted trajectory. This has been the case partly due to the complex and elusive nature of mental health conditions and partly to the problematic status of psychiatry in relation to medical sciences. The (relative) success of psychotropic drugs, the development and widespread use of brain neuroimaging techniques, and advances in genetics have stimulated in recent years the search for biomarkers for mental health conditions and have contributed to the proliferation and diversification of professionals working in this field. Nevertheless, mental health expertise continues to be challenged, with some critics denouncing it for pathologizing variations in average human behavior (Horwitz & Wakefield, 2007), and others condemning it for medicalizing social and political problems (Metzl, 2009). Furthermore, people diagnosed have assumed an increasingly active role in the production of knowledge about mental health, and not always in collaboration with medical professionals. Given the tremendous increase of mental health diagnoses around the world (Rose, 2018), it is more important than ever to understand how expertise about mental health is currently performed online, by whom, and through what means.

This book addresses these issues by focusing on bipolar disorder, a mental health condition which has become more prominent over the last few decades, and which is currently among the top ten causes of disability worldwide (Whiteford et al., 2013). It is a mood disorder characterized by the alternation of depressive and manic episodes and marked by episode-free intervals. While it is thought to be determined by a combination of neurological, genetic, and environmental factors, the precise causes of this condition are currently unknown. It is studied by various specialists: psychiatrists,   psychologists,   neuroscientists, endocrinologists, molecular biologists, epidemiologists, and so on. These professionals focus on different sites as the origin and location of this condition, they use different techniques and materials, and so they understand rather different things by bipolar disorder (Dehue, 2008; Hacking, 1995; Mol, 2002). Furthermore, the therapeutic approaches used for its management consist of diverse combinations of chemical substances, talk and behavioral therapies, as well as technological interventions, such as transcranial magnetic stimulation or vagus nerve stimulation. Dominant approaches in personalized medicine have further enhanced the complexity characterizing this field, as new subgroups have been distinguished among the people diagnosed with this condition based on whether or not they exhibited specific genetic modifications, and on their responses to certain medications. Furthermore, these perspectives shape and are shaped by the ways in which people diagnosed with this condition experience it. Bipolar disorder can therefore be seen as a "moving target" (Hacking, 1999), since it mobilizes different types of knowledge, groups of professionals, tools, standards, and methods in dynamic configurations. This makes the study of this condition relevant for research on expertise, as it can lead to a better understanding of the ways in which expertise is performed when numerous factors are involved and when a field is marked by numerous known as well as unknown unknowns.

Expertise about mental health has been traditionally performed in the hallways of medical institutions, in laboratories and clinics, and on the pages of compendia and scientific journals. However, since the late 1990s, when the Internet began to be widely adopted, the prominence of this medium as a new site for the provision of knowledge and the performance of expertise has grown (Fox et al., 2005; Hardey, 1999; Hu & Sundar, 2010). This has been particularly the case after the development of Web 2.0 technologies, such as social media platforms and wikis, where people could not only consume mental health-related information, but also actively engage in its production. As medical information has become accessible to broad audiences and as people diagnosed have started to play a more active role in the development of knowledge, some scholars thought that the Internet would contribute to more equal or balanced relationships between medical professionals and people diagnosed, what some (Kitcher, 2011; Topol, 2015) have referred to as "democratization." While more nuanced studies have since been provided (Kivits, 2009; Versteeg & Te Molder, 2018; Ziebland & Wyke, 2012) and while people diagnosed increasingly use digital technologies for various health-related purposes, it is yet unclear what exactly the latter contribute and how these contributions are used. Nor are there many results available on the ways in which the Internet has shaped how "traditional" experts perform expertise. This study contributes to these discussions by asking how different stakeholders use the Internet to perform expertise and how democratizing such practices are. Furthermore, by combining insights from media studies on different types of online encounters and their dynamic character with sociological perspectives on the potential of personalized and precision medicine for the development of new types of communities (Akrich, 2010; Stommel & Lamerichs, 2014; Tutton & Prainsack, 2011), this book explores the possibility of new individual-group configurations in the online performance of expertise about bipolar disorder.

Despite attempts to stabilize expertise about mental health, knowledge about mental health conditions is not universal, but depends on the social, cultural, and economic contexts in which it is made manifest (Kleinman, 1988; Lakoff, 2005). Thus, how bipolar disorder is recognized, understood, and intervened upon depends on the ways in which the provision of mental healthcare is organized in any given country, and on the interpretative tools used by professionals. It is also informed by the different ways in which people learn to distinguish and make sense of problematic experiences from the incessant flow of physical and psychological stimuli and reactions that make up their lives. This raises important questions about the fate of such local and cultural markers in the online performance of expertise about bipolar disorder. To cast some light onto these aspects, this study compares the American and French perspectives on bipolar disorder and use of online technologies in mental healthcare. Given the growing popularity of online platforms among people diagnosed with mental health conditions (Carron-Arthur et al., 2016; Naslund et al., 2016), such findings are very important, because cultural and social elements may influence who feels entitled to share information, what type of information is shared, and how it is subsequently interpreted and put to use by readers. In an attempt to avoid cultural reification, the results of such comparison are presented at the level of each chapter, thus illustrating how various similarities and differences developed as an integral part of the specific analyses conducted.

Over the coming chapters we will see that the performance of expertise about bipolar disorder is not a straightforward process by which offline practices, tools, and approaches are transferred online, but involves additional skills and complex negotiations, which sometimes lead to unexpected configurations. The analysis of the empirical materials collected prompted the realization that the current theoretical perspectives on expertise do not sufficiently account for the complexity of positions that relevant stakeholders occupy and for the different types of relations they need to cultivate to successfully contribute to the development of expertise. That is why I put forward a new approach to expertise, wherein expertise is conceived as a practical achievement, realized through coordination and affective labor among stakeholders who occupy multiple and shifting positions across a complex ecosystem (discussed in more detail later in this chapter). This new approach is arrived at by engaging in dialogue with and building upon influential theories on expertise in STS. In the process, several empirical and theoretical contributions are made. Building on STS insights on users, this book contributes to medical sociology by showing that through their specific engagement with the online affordances of blogs and fora, people diagnosed with bipolar disorder move beyond the performance of lay expertise, and put forward what I call "digitally enabled hypotheses" about treatment effectiveness (Chap. 3). By bringing insights from media studies in dialogue with the recently developed field of Studies of Expertise and Experience (SEE), the concept of interactional expertise developed by Collins and Evans (2002) is expanded in this book by taking into consideration the effects of the medium through which it is performed (Chap. 5). At a time when the current dominant neoliberal model of governance encourages people to take up behaviors illustrative of narrowly conceived notions of individual autonomy and personal responsibility, we will see that some people diagnosed with bipolar disorder follow up on such encouragements and use the Internet to become successful entrepreneurs (Chap. 5), while others develop more nuanced approaches, performing solidarity and contributing to the collective development of lay expertise together with others with whom they share important similarities (Chap. 6).

In the remainder of this chapter, I discuss the details of the research upon which this book draws and introduce the following chapters. I begin, however, with an overview of the main sociological approaches to the study of expertise.

Theoretical Approaches to Expertise

Expertise means different things to different people, it is performed differently in different contexts, and it leads to different relations between people who hold expertise and those who do not as well as between those endowed with different types of expertise. While the Oxford Dictionary first mentions the term "expertise" in 1869, it was not until the 1970s that expertise started to gain considerable academic interest, thereby "reflect[ing] the growth and proliferation of professions with specialized forms of knowledge, and (…) the increased commodification of knowledge production" (McNeil, 1998: 56-57). It has thus far mainly been studied within the fields of psychology, philosophy, and sociology (Young & Muller, 2014), and such forays have been characterized by important disciplinary differences as well as significant distinctions in approach and conceptualization at the level of each discipline broadly understood (Williams et al., 1998) (for a discussion of the main approaches to expertise in psychology and philosophy, see Annex 1). Realist and constructivist approaches to expertise can be noted in all these fields. According to realist perspectives, expertise is a real and substantive skill that certain people possess. Constructivist approaches see expertise as attributional, as a qualification that experts enjoy based on it having been granted to them by others who have the prerogative to do so and which is subsequently socially recognized. Further distinctions can be derived from these two main perspectives, such as whether expertise is the property of individuals or groups, and whether it is primarily a form of theoretical or practical knowledge.

In sociology, expertise has initially been studied from the perspective of the sociology of professions, with early studies seeking to understand what accounted for the differences between occupations and professions (Kotzee, 2014). The focus has therefore been mainly on expertise as a property of groups, developed through various processes of acculturation. Initially, a realist view of expertise seems to have dominated sociological studies, with various authors showing the differences between professions and occupations to be substantial and even providing various lists of characteristics for each of them (Evetts et al., 2006). In time, however, as the constructivist approach to expertise has come to dominate (Koppl, 2010), these authors have been criticized for helping maintain the authority of influential professions, such as medicine and law (Saks, 2012). Such critique is in line with (neo)Marxist perspectives which conceive of expertise as a social construction, as a means through which influential groups retain a monopoly over certain services, with professional training, standards, and evaluations seen as mechanisms through which outsiders of these groups are denied access (Illich, 1977; Susskind & Susskind, 2015). Building upon such insights, feminist and postcolonial scholars have denounced the close relation between knowledge, authority, and power, and have shown the tenuous links between expertise, ethnicity, and gender, among others. From this perspective, rather than something real, based upon substantial ability in a given field, expertise is seen as an attribute bestowed upon certain members of society by specific institutions, but which has real and important consequences in terms of the distribution of power and privileges.

The debate regarding the contribution of STS scholars to the charges currently brought against expertise in "post-truth" discussions is still ongoing (Collins et al., 2017; Fuller, 2017; Lynch, 2017; Radder, 2018; Sismondo, 2017), but there is no doubt that they have been important proponents and advocates of the constructivist view on expertise. For instance, influential studies in the field (and in the sociology of scientific knowledge) have revealed how political and social considerations shape the production of scientific knowledge (Barnes, 1974; Bijker, 1995; Bloor, 1976; Shapin & Schaffer, 1985). In STS, currently, three main approaches can be distinguished in the study of expertise. The first highlights the substantial character of expertise and challenges the idea that public engagement means that all views are equal, represented by Collins and Evans (2002, 2007). The second conceives of expertise in terms of its institutional embedding and is put forward by Jasanoff (2004). The third understands expertise as a property of discrete networks, and it was developed by Eyal and colleagues in their study on autism (Eyal, 2013; Eyal et al., 2010; Eyal & Hart, 2010).

Seeking to determine the bases upon which members of different communities could be involved in decision-making processes at various levels depending on the type of knowledge they were endowed with, Collins and Evans (2007) put forward the Periodic Table of Expertise. In their view, expertise is characterized by three dimensions: esotericity, or the degree to which expertise is confined to a particular group; the tacit knowledge required for it; and the changes in expert performance, which trace a novice's trajectory as s/he becomes a member of the expert group. Given the topic of this book, it has been helpful to engage with Collins and Evans' insights, as on the one hand they have tried to open up the concept of expertise by acknowledging that people without official accreditations could also be experts in a given field, while on the other they have sought to ensure that expertise continues to designate something "real" (Collins & Evans, 2007:40). Particularly useful has been the distinction between what they call "contributory" and "interactional expertise," which Collins and Evans consider specialist forms of expertise requiring specialist tacit knowledge. While they conceptualize contributory expertise as the ability to contribute productively to a field, interactional expertise refers to the ability to become fluent in the language of practice of a given domain, thereby being able to engage in substantial discussions about relevant matters with contributory experts in that field (I discuss at length this form of expertise in Chap. 5). Thus, Collins and Evans' conceptualization focuses on expertise as a matter of one's knowledge and competence.

While this approach is meant to fight relativism, it neglects the strong relational undertones of expertise, as it is acquired, maintained, and displayed in complex and often long-lasting exchanges between people with different levels of knowledge of a field and with different stakes in it. Even though Collins and Evans' typology of expertise is fruitfully applied in this book, it is important to note some of the criticism it has received. Jasanoff (2004), for example, views expertise as embedded in practice, that is, as enacted in specific institutional settings, and she has reproached Collins and Evans for not having sufficiently taken into account the role of national and institutional cultures in shaping the development and content of expertise and the relations between experts and society at large. Jasanoff argues that socio-political elements play an important role in determining what counts as authoritative knowledge and in ensuring the obduracy of such understandings (Jasanoff, 2004), be they more or less well-founded. These elements ascribe authority and credibility, indicating who the public should trust and defer to in specific matters. Thus, according to Jasanoff (2003:393), "expertise is not merely something that is in the heads and hands of skilled persons, constituted through their deep familiarity with the problem in question, but rather [...] it is something acquired, and deployed, within particular historical, political, and cultural contexts."

Whereas Jasanoff conceives of expertise as grounded in institutions, Eyal has put forward an understanding of expertise as "a network linking together agents, devices, concepts, and institutional and spatial arrangements" (Eyal, 2013: 863). Building upon insights put forward by Foucault (1972/2010) and Rose (1992), Eyal finds it important to distinguish between expertise and experts, arguing that the study of each requires different methods and casts light upon different aspects. In this understanding, expertise is not the attribute of any one individual, but it is distributed, coming into being through exchanges between "agents" endowed with different abilities and insights yet committed to solving a common issue through similar methods. Eyal developed this theory studying how the parents of autistic children challenged the psychiatric establishment and succeeded in putting forward a different understanding of this condition and in popularizing a new therapeutic approach. These transformations were set into motion, in Eyal's view, by a checklist that an army psychiatrist, book author, and parent of an autistic child, Bernard Rimland, provided on the back of his book for the parents of autistic children to fill in and send back to him. Thus, the checklist represented an innovative model of knowledge exchange around which the network was organized, a means which allowed new stakeholders to contribute actively to the production of knowledge about autism. His distinction between experts and expertise allows Eyal to conclude that while psychiatrists may have lost in this way some of their territory, as we will also see in Chap. 2, psychiatric expertise was in fact expanded in that it became part of a greater network, consisting of more domains and institutions and touching upon broader areas of life. Expertise as a network implies a variable level of flexibility, as it may be more or less easily rewired depending on the different stakeholder's resources, skills, and creativity, on the credibility they enjoy, and on the necessity to develop new goals.

This conceptualization of expertise resonates with insights put forward by scholars working in different fields in response to the highly complex, dynamic, and interconnected world we live in. Important here are the insights provided by Edwards (2010), working in the field of professional learning, in reaction to the realization that people with expertise in a given field are increasingly required to work outside the boundaries of their particular institutions, to perform their expertise in collaboration with specialists from different fields, with different training, methodologies, and perspectives on the issues at hand. She argues that these realities have led to a "relational turn in expertise" (2010), as they require "an expertise which includes recognising and responding to the standpoints of others and is in addition to the specialist knowledge at the core of each distinct professional practice" (Edwards, 2010:2). Edwards thus seems to believe that such social skills have now become necessary at a more general level rather than being required only for some types of expertise (Kotzee, 2014). While it is indebted to Collins and Evans' notion of interactional expertise, this perspective has the merit of seeking to move toward a more collective and dynamic understanding of expertise.

Edwards' understanding of expertise resonates with a more recent contribution from education and communication studies, where Engeström (2018) has argued in favor of the need to transition to a "collaborative and transformative expertise." Expertise derives then from common activities undertaken by different types of practitioners, who are flexible, open to new knowledge, and capable of dealing with rapidly changing environments. Particularly relevant for this book is Engeström's (2018:1) argument that "[c]ollaborative and transformative medical expertise is continuous negotiation and hybridization of the insights of medical professionals and their patients. Without patients' insights, accounts, and actions, medical expertise would at best be merely top-down engineering." Rather than approaching expertise as an outstanding performance, Engeström studies it "as everyday work" by focusing on mundane situations when disturbances, breakdowns, and/or rapid transformations interrupt daily routine. What is particularly interesting about his approach is that he takes a collective activity as a unit of analysis for expertise and considers it not only a matter of internalizing authoritative knowledge, but also as conducive to new ways to produce and manifest knowledge

Building upon the relational aspect of expertise in a different way, Kotzee and Smit (2017), philosophers of science, tried to reconcile realist and constructivist views by putting forward a new conceptualization. Their starting point is the realization that both perspectives conceive of expertise as relational: in the first case, expertise is seen as consisting of the relationship between an individual and an ability; in the second, it consists of the relationship between an individual and others who acknowledge him/her as an expert in a given domain. Their solution relies on combining these elements to define expertise as one's "ability and/or level of knowledge…that significantly surpasses [that of others]" (Kotzee & Smit, 2017:647). Given the highly specialized world in which we live, knowing whose opinion to ask for and whose advice to trust on a specific issue is highly necessary, and expertise thus understood fulfills an important public function. Nevertheless, Kotzee and Smit fail to consider a third type of relationship, namely that which people with expertise in a field develop with others who hold expertise in a different field. The analytical movement between these perspectives on expertise and the empirical materials collected for the study described in this book highlighted the fact that this concept could be further refined, especially in light of the transformations brought about by digitalization. It is to the new approach to expertise that thus emerged that I now turn.

A New Approach to Expertise

The engagement with theoretical perspectives on expertise and with the empirical materials led to a new working definition of expertise, where expertise is understood as a practical achievement, realized though coordination and affective labor among stakeholders who occupy multiple and shifting positions across a complex ecosystem. Through this definition I position myself among scholars who take a constructivist as well as practice-oriented approach to expertise in ways which I briefly describe below.

This definition is vastly indebted to Mol's (2002) concept of enactment, as the articulation and making manifest of substantial knowledge and abilities through complex entanglements of people and tools are also essential elements in this new conceptualization. Thus, the main difference between her perspective and the one developed here may be seen as a shift in focus dictated by the societal changes and practical transformations that have taken place in recent years. Mol put forward the concept of enactment because it allowed her to make clear that the distinction between human subjects and natural objects is blurred: "like (human) subjects, (natural) objects are framed as part of events that occur and plays that are staged. If an object is real this is because it is part of a practice. It is a reality *enacted*" (Mol, 2002:44, emphasis in the original). I share with Mol the concern to foreground the multiplicity of the object resulting from such practices, but I add to her perspective the emphasis on the numerous, fragmented, and dynamic identities of the actors involved, to use her terminology. These were not sufficiently considered, since her account focused mainly on the professional identity of the medical professionals studied, although some intimations thereof can be noted in her discussion of the life of "patients" outside the medical setting. Enactments or performances thus grant people and objects "fragile identities" (Mol, 2002), which may shift from one site to the other.

Mol's perspective is combined in this new understanding of expertise with the insights developed by Engeström (2018), in particular his emphasis on the collective, dynamic, and adaptable character of expertise in current times. According to Engeström (2018), expertise requires both vertical and horizontal types of movement, as knowledge in a given area needs not only to be deepened, but has to be enriched with knowledge from other related areas. By combining this perspective on the dynamic character of expertise with Jasanoff's (2004) call to pay attention to the cultural and institutional elements that shape it, the understanding of expertise as an achievement across a complex ecosystem emerged. This conceptualization prompts the analysts to look beyond the practices they may be observing, to broaden their focus to include perspectives on the rights and obligations of the different stakeholders involved, on the prevailing cultural norms and expectations about their activities. Thus, how expertise is performed constitutes both an illustration of and a reaction to specific historical developments, to legal, political, and educational provisions and to the future visions animating the field at a given moment in time. For instance, new legal provisions about the acceptability of certain digital practices and the use of online data may enable and deter people diagnosed with bipolar disorder to share their insights and seek to engage in epistemic practices using digital technologies.

Edwards' (2010) views on relational expertise have highlighted the necessity for different types of professionals or stakeholders to work together in order to achieve a common goal, but Engeström (2018) sets the threshold somewhat lower by foregrounding coordination rather than agreement. This means that the stakeholders involved need not undergo a substantial transformation and come to share the same understanding of the various concepts, processes, and tools involved, nor do they have to use the same standards. What is important is that they agree to suspend their differences in order to achieve a common goal (a minimal form of agreement) under conditions of uncertainty and, often, within a limited time frame. Thus, one of the advantages of "coordination" in relation to expertise is that it does not emphasize the epistemic differences between individuals in regard to a specific topic or domain, which, for instance, Kotzee and Smit's (2017) conceptualization highlights. It foregrounds, instead, the development of more similar and equal (temporary) relations, thereby shifting the focus from people who have and do not have substantial abilities and knowledge in a field to the interactions between people who may be equally endowed, but in other domains, and who may have to work together to solve complex problems.

This perspective is further indebted to psychological and philosophical perspectives on expertise, which highlight the importance of affective reactions in relation to the development of expertise and argue that highly competent people not only come to know things differently, but also to feel differently toward them (Dreyfus & Dreyfus, 1986; Selinger & Crease, 2006). While these perspectives mainly focus on the affective responses an individual may have in relation to the practices at which s/he is (becoming) an expert, the online interactions that will be described in this book highlight the numerous emotions that arise and need to be managed when different people interact and share insights online. These emotions played an important role in the development of new knowledge online, as interactions among people diagnosed could be short or longer-lasting, superficial, or more substantial, depending on the emotions that dominated such encounters, which shaped, in turn, the insights that were shared. Thus, to perform lay expertise online, some people diagnosed had to overcome their fright or reservations regarding computers and the Internet, they had to try to make themselves likeable or intriguing enough for others to interact with them, and they had to care for others, to respect their views and experiences and to help them develop more positive emotions. This means that expertise is not solely a matter of intellectual and cognitive processes, but that affective labor plays an important part in its development, as it underlies people's efforts to coordinate with others.

The focus on the multiple and shifting positions that stakeholders can occupy in relation to the development of expertise is indebted to feminist theories (Harding, 2004), which have emphasized the different meanings an issue can acquire depending on the perspective of those who look upon it, on the identity and position they occupy within a certain social order. While Richmond (2017) has suggested to approach expertise by considering the mediation work individuals or groups at the periphery are forced to undertake in order to (effectively) communicate with those at the center, her discussion of Lugones' concept of "mobile positioning" has been particularly useful here. Thus, by paying attention to the multiple identities one inhabits, one may find ways to escape, obfuscate, resist, or transform the norms and regulations of the communities one is part of, and one may develop a more critical perspective on them. This informed the realization that one and the same stakeholder may occupy different positions within the ecosystem where expertise is developed and that these different positionings may need to be both "stirred" and managed at different moments throughout this process. For instance, in the field of mental health, numerous researchers, and medical professionals are also patients or carers and fulfill executive functions whereby they contribute to the decision-making regarding the allocation of research funds.

The new insights that can be acquired by applying this new understanding of expertise will be illustrated throughout the findings described in each chapter. Since expertise is a practical achievement in a complex ecosystem, the important role of historical developments and future visions in animating the epistemic efforts of various stakeholders will be brought to the fore in Chap. 2, while the ways in which expertise is shaped by dominant social values will be discussed in Chap. 6. Chapters 3 and 4 will highlight two dimensions of coordination, both of which are mediated in different ways by the design and affordances of digital platforms. Whereas Chap. 3 focuses on the material and epistemic relations that one and the same stakeholder needs to develop and maintain across different digital spaces to successfully perform expertise, Chap. 4 shows that digital technologies inform coordination in substantial ways by allowing for the coming together of disparate efforts undertaken by many, sometimes fleeting, contributors. The multiple and shifting positions that stakeholders can occupy in relation to expertise will be brought to the fore across Chaps. 4 and 5, as it will be shown how some individuals diagnosed with bipolar disorder manage to position themselves as experts by experience, representatives of people diagnosed with bipolar disorder, patients, advisors, and successful entrepreneurs. As we will see, it is their successful orchestration of these multiple identities and their ability to shift the focus from one to the other, depending on the character of their interactions and of their goals, that have enabled them to become highly influential. While affective practices could be encountered across all the online exchanges studied, they will come to the fore in Chap. 6, where it will be argued that affective labor shapes the development of expertise as it contributes to the development of new collectives and facilitates the exchange of intensely intimate experiences about bipolar disorder.

As it must have become clear by now, the concept of performance, first introduced by Goffman (1959/1990), was used to investigate expertise about bipolar disorder on digital platforms. According to Goffman, social interactions represent performances through which individuals seek to produce desired impressions on their audiences by engaging in various practices of self-revelation and concealment. Even though some scholars (Barad, 2003) have understood performance in a very limited way, as something akin to engaging in an activity, whereas others (Mol, 2002) have preferred the notion of "enactment" which did not carry within it the implicit distinction between a real self/"persona" or inner identity versus a "mask" or external identity, this concept is used here in a broader sense, which highlights the important coordination required for a particular version of reality (Hafermalz et al., 2016) to be brought into being. Given the focus on practices, materialities, and events that it allows for, performance was deemed appropriate in view of the new conceptualization of expertise put forward. This way, the impact of the Internet and its multifaceted character on epistemic practices can be brought to the fore, as expertise about bipolar disorder can be approached as being distributed across different online platforms, and shaped by the different technologies available on them. Before moving on to that, however, there are still a few elements which need to be introduced, namely bipolar disorder and the role of the Internet in the study of expertise about this condition, to which I now turn.

Bipolar Disorder

Mental health conditions are the result of complex interactions between individuals with a certain biological make-up and their physical and social environment. Symptoms of what would later be known as bipolar disorder were first presented in the 1850s to the *Académie de Medicine* in Paris by Baillarger, who called it *"folie à double forme"* (dual form insanity), and Falret, who referred to it as *"folie circulaire"* (circular insanity) (Angst & Sellaro, 2000). Both scientists agreed that this condition had a terrible prognosis, and Falret postulated that it had a strong genetic basis. In the 1900s, Kraepelin was also pessimistic about the outcome of patients exhibiting such symptoms, but observed that they also experienced intervals when no "abnormal" functioning could be detected. He used the term "manic-depressive psychosis" to distinguish this mood condition from "precocious madness," which later became known as schizophrenia (Angst & Marneros, 2001). The term "manic-depressive illness" was coined in the 1950s, which roughly coincides with the period when lithium salts started their successful, still ongoing career as treatment for this condition, following a discovery by Australian psychiatrist John Cade (Healy, 2008). In the 1980s, the name was replaced by "bipolar disorder," thought to be less stigmatizing, but this change continues to be debated, as many medical professionals and people diagnosed consider the former denomination to convey the character of this condition more appropriately.

Currently, the presumed causes of bipolar disorder represent a mixture of neurologic, genetic, and environmental factors, and this condition is managed through a combination of medication, therapy, and counseling. Because of the similarity in symptoms with major depression, bipolar disorder remains difficult to diagnose correctly, and often many years (5–12) and numerous encounters with various mental health professionals are necessary. In the Diagnostic and Statistical Manual of Mental Disorders (DSM-5, 2013), this condition is coded as bipolar single manic, bipolar manic, bipolar depressed, bipolar mixed, each category containing several subtypes. The International Classification of Disease and Health Related Problems (ICD-10, 2010) groups conditions based on their relatedness to each other, so different forms of bipolar disorder are spread under the headings of various types of mental health conditions. An important distinction both in regard to diagnostic difficulties but also in relation to treatment lies between the types bipolar I disorder and bipolar II disorder. These two types differ mainly in the severity of the manic episodes experienced. Whereas bipolar I disorder involves severe manic episodes, lasting for several days and at times requiring hospitalization, those diagnosed with bipolar II disorder experience hypomanic states rather than full-blown manic episodes (Grande et al., 2016). Even though the enormous increase in people diagnosed is often ascribed to improved diagnostic tools, it may also be due to a positive re-evaluation of this condition. Martin (2009), for example, argues this is the result of a close connection between the values of capitalism and some of the traits associated with manic episodes: creativity, passion, dedication, and intense activity. In contrast, others have explained the growing number of people diagnosed with this condition by arguing that the values of capitalism lead to stress, anxiety, and depression (Hidaka, 2012), while yet others have linked this increase to tendencies to medicalize social issues (Esposito & Perez, 2014) and to pathologize variations in human experiences (Horwitz & Wakefield, 2007; Scott, 2006).

Bipolar disorder has also been affected by recent developments in personalized and precision medicine, which provide visions of medical interventions tailored to the specific needs and circumstances of individuals (Rose, 2018). Doubts about the scientific character of expertise about mental health have led professionals to embrace perspectives and procedures which have deeply anchored this condition in biology, in processes which could be identified, measured, and acted upon through targeted approaches. As such, in the aftermath of the Human Genome Project (1990–2003), numerous research projects (Alda et al., 2005; Cruceanu et al., 2009; MacQueen et al., 2001) have been undertaken, which have sought to identify the phenotypes and genetic markers underlying bipolar disorder, the predictive factors of response among different (sub) groups of people diagnosed, and new drug targets. At present, however, bipolar disorder seems to be characterized by too great genetic and phenotypic heterogeneity for these insights to be very helpful (Rose, 2018). Furthermore, since treatment response in many of these studies was measured with different instruments, the translation of these new insights into clinical practice is likely to take some time and to require collaboration and intense efforts among a very broad range of professionals, including not only medical specialists but also engineers and computer scientists.

Even though DSM-5 and ICD-10 largely determine how mental health conditions are diagnosed around the world, expertise about them is shaped by the social and cultural context of its performance. To better understand the role these elements play, this book focuses on expertise about bipolar disorder in the US and France. These countries were chosen because their approach to mental healthcare is marked by a diverse range of similarities and differences, which can better highlight the role the Internet plays in mediating them. Thus, whereas both countries are in the process of reforming their mental healthcare system, there remain notable differences between them regarding the diagnosis and management of mental health conditions. In France, mental disorders are diagnosed based on ICD-10 and a psychosocial model of disease remains prevalent, whereas in the US diagnosis is based on DSM-5 and the focus is on the biological markers of this condition. There are also important differences regarding the number of people diagnosed with bipolar disorder among the two countries, as the US registers the highest number of people diagnosed in the world, with an incidence of 4%, whereas in France, the rate is significantly lower, with 1.5–2% of the population being diagnosed.[1] While bipolar disorder is generally thought to affect both genders equally, the results of the most recent French national survey suggest that bipolar disorder is starting to become a gendered condition here, as the statistics indicate that there are 1.6 times more women diagnosed than men, the difference concerning specifically bipolar disorder type II (Vaugrente, 2018). In both countries, however, stigma remains rampant, despite the efforts undertaken by various advocacy movements, which will be briefly discussed in the next chapter. At the same time, both the US and France share an interest in using telemedicine and digital technologies for the provision of mental healthcare. Since the Internet is an important carrier of social and cultural markers (Miller & Slater, 2000; Orgad, 2005), studying how expertise about bipolar disorder is performed on digital platforms by contributors from both countries is therefore highly relevant, and it is this aspect that I now briefly discuss.

---

[1] The exact numbers may differ depending on the studies consulted and on the forms of bipolar disorder included.

Studying Expertise About Bipolar Disorder Online

While the Internet is intensively used these days for health-related purposes, it continues to divide opinions about the ways in which it shapes (mental) healthcare, and about the benefits and disadvantages of its use for different stakeholders. Thus, its proponents, many of which are government officials, argue that it may help solve the current crisis in mental healthcare, brought about by a growing number of people diagnosed and lower budget funds available for this sector, as it may enable the provision of good quality and cost-effective care. These optimistic views have acquired renewed impetus with the move toward personalized and precision medicine and with the hopes generated by big data analytics. These have changed the ways in which health and disease are conceptualized and have emphasized the need for (self)surveillance and for collecting highly diverse types of data both from people diagnosed and from those not (yet) diagnosed (Hogle, 2016; Prainsack, 2018). In this context, active forms of patienthood have been encouraged not only by public stakeholders, but also by commercial actors, which have started to become more involved in healthcare (Sharon, 2016), as we shall see in the next chapter.

Critics (Brown & Baker, 2012; Lupton, 2018; Neff, 2013) have argued, however, that such approaches constitute strategies through which governments place greater responsibilities upon citizens in a context where social provisions are cut and where a market logic is increasingly used to guide the provision of mental healthcare. Some commentators have also criticized the users' engagement with digital technologies as a form of free labor (Mitchell & Waldby, 2010; Terranova, 2000; Waldby & Cooper, 2008), where people are encouraged to constantly monitor themselves in pervasive and invasive ways, but are required to give up ownership over their data and any claims over potential profits that can be made from them. Others have also worried about the different ways in which such data may be used and how they may affect the individual users of such technologies and the prescription practices of medical professionals. Such concerns are particularly well-founded in the US, where Section 2713 of the Affordable Care Act stipulates the establishment of "guidelines to permit a health insurance plan to use value-based insurance design" (National Conference of State Legislatures, 2018). Thus, while some believe the Internet can be harnessed to help solve numerous problems in mental healthcare, others worry about the effects of online practices, about the ways in which people diagnosed understand themselves and their condition, and about the ways in which the Internet can shape relations between them and medical professionals. This book contributes toward a better understanding of these aspects by engaging with two recurrent ideas about the Internet's potential, namely its ability to democratize and to help transmit local and cultural norms.

In the early days of the Internet, some medical sociologists and media scholars thought that it would contribute to the democratization of relations between medical professionals and their patients (Hardey, 1999; Poster, 2001) by allowing people diagnosed to access medical information previously reserved strictly for medical professionals, by enabling them to learn about alternative approaches to mental health, and by facilitating their contributions to epistemic practices. In the meantime, more nuanced studies (Nettleton & Burrows, 2003; Wyatt et al., 2016) have been published, which have problematized the Internet's democratizing potential, highlighting the multifaceted character of this medium, and the heterogeneity of people who search for and contribute to health-related information online. Scholars have also argued that the Internet leads to new forms of inequality engendered by various algorithms, including those of search engines, which determine the visibility of digital platforms (Bishop, 2018; Hargittai, 2007; Pasquinelli, 2009).

The resources available to people are thus not equally distributed, as online communication skills, familiarity with various technologies, and the size and impact of on- and offline (professional) networks can differ considerably. Furthermore, despite their increasing popularity, interactive digital platforms have not replaced non-interactive websites, but co-exist with them. The choice of an interactive or non-interactive platform is determined not only by the goals and preferences of users, but also by their resources and position. Thus, important institutions with a generous budget can invest in their platform, but need to shape the information provided in view of their values. In contrast, smaller stake-holders may need to settle for a platform they can afford or select a design that will attract many visitors, and attune their message to the (prospective) sponsors' preferences. These choices may affect a platform's index score with a search engine, which can have profound consequences, as studies about people's online search behavior indicate that users often do not look beyond the first few results pages (Bar-Ilan et al., 2006; Höchstötter & Lewandowski, 2009). Thus, the type of platform selected and its design significantly influence how information is provided, and the types of knowledge made available.

In the early days, the Internet was also seen by some scholars as an instrument of globalization, as they believed that it would help bring about cultural homogeneity through the seamless flow of information among people from all corners of the world and through the subsequent effacement of local practices in favor of cosmopolitan approaches (Featherstone et al., 1995). After 2000, however, a growing number of anthropologists and media scholars have drawn attention to the specific contexts in which online contributions are made, and have argued that social and cultural norms importantly shape people's online behaviors (Ardichvili et al., 2006; Fox et al., 2005; Miller & Slater, 2000). Yet little is currently known about the ways in which local and cultural markers shape online exchanges about mental health, and this is one of the aspects that this study addresses by comparing how expertise about bipolar disorder is performed on American and French platforms. In so doing, it focuses on the ways in which online contributors from these countries use different digital platforms and the affordances available on them to determine how local perspectives shape people's orientations toward bipolar disorder online. More details about the methodological approaches used are provided below.

Methods and Sources

Methodologically, this book draws upon qualitative empirical material of two types: data collected from different digital platforms on bipolar disorder and articles from medical journals. Digital platforms are spaces which are socially created through interactions and practices between numerous stakeholders. They can be endowed with different affordances, and require different levels of skills and resources by their users (Drucker, 2011). Affordances denote mechanisms which are conceptually relational and which place different opportunities and constraints on both users and artifacts (Davis & Chouinard, 2016). This means that not all platforms and functions embedded on them are equally accessible to all users. Online contributions are therefore informed not only by the availability or absence of various functions, such as the ability to comment and to upload texts, graphs, images, and videos, but also by the users' skills, preferences, and attitudes toward these technologies as well as by what they hope to achieve through their sharing practices. The advent of Web 2.0 has heightened the profile of interactive platforms, which are characterized by a high media convergence (Herring, 2012), meaning that information is increasingly provided through a combination of text with other visual, audio, and video materials. Yet, such platforms exist in an environment that they share with non-interactive platforms, which are less dynamic, complex, and open. Non-interactive platforms dedicated to mental health generally include websites belonging to influential institutions, be they governmental bodies, or patient organizations, which importantly shape the provision of treatment and care for people diagnosed with bipolar disorder. While the access to the information they provide is public, the contributors are selected by each particular institution and are generally medical professionals.

In order to understand how the Internet shapes the performance of expertise about bipolar disorder, both interactive and non-interactive online platforms were selected. The selection was based upon a novel methodological approach, as I aimed to reproduce the behavior of average Internet users and conducted queries using the index of the search engine Google as a relevance indicator. A list was thus made of the online platforms mentioned on the first 30 pages of results. This list was subsequently filtered to exclude online platforms in other languages than English and French, to eliminate multiple pointers to the same item and websites where the content was not focused on bipolar disorder or which were not free to access, but required registration or payment. Since language is not a reliable indicator, the domain of each platform was subsequently checked and only the online platforms were retained where American and French official institutions were mentioned. This was done to ensure that online data were collected from contributors in these two countries. Blogs and fora which had been established for less than one year at the moment when the selection took place (September 2014), which did not allow the information available on their platforms to be used for research purposes, and which had few contributors (<10) were also filtered out.

The table below gives an overview of the online platforms from which data were collected:

List of selected platforms for data collection

Platform name and country	Platform type	Platform management
National Institute of Mental Health—US	Non-interactive	Governmental agency
Bipolar Burble—US	Blog	Person diagnosed
Bipolar Happens!—US	Blog	Person diagnosed
Bp Hope—US	Forum	People diagnosed
La Haute Autorité de Santé (HAS)—France	Non-interactive	Governmental agency
Doctissimo—France	Forum	People diagnosed; mediated by medical professionals
Le Forum des Bipotes—France	Forum	People diagnosed

Data were collected at different moments between June 2014 and September 2018, because online contributors often change their mind about the online reactions they provide and amend them (multiple times) or remove them altogether at later moments. By collecting the data from the same platforms in different periods, it was possible to identify instances when comments had been edited or removed by the people who had written them and thus to respect their wishes by removing them from the data collected. These data were supplemented by the collection of newspaper and digital articles and communications (Chap. 2), relevant medical articles (Chap. 4), and online interviews with two highly influential bloggers on bipolar disorder (Chap. 5). To understand how expertise about bipolar disorder was performed on these different online platforms and how meaning and culture were (re)produced online, qualitative methods which could provide "deep knowledge" of such dynamic and situated practices (Markham, 2016) were used. The specific methods used in each chapter vary, but they include computer-mediated discourse analysis (Chap. 4), thematic analysis (Chaps. 3, 5, and 6), and conversation analysis (Chap. 6) adapted to online contexts.

The approval of the Ethical Review Committee Inner City (ERCIC) of Maastricht University was sought and obtained on April 6, 2016. It was not feasible to obtain informed consent from all the online contributors who posted information on the platforms from which data were. This was partly due to their sheer number and partly due to the fact that the contributions collected span roughly 10 years, a period in which many people who shared their insights may have stopped using these platforms or may have changed their usernames. Since data were collected from platforms with a public character, the study upon which this book is based meets current ethical guidelines for online research. For instance, according to the British Psychological Society (BPS, 2013:7), "where it is reasonable to argue that there is likely no perception and/or expectation of privacy (or where scientific/social value and/or research validity considerations are deemed to justify undisclosed observation), use of research data without gaining valid consent may be justifiable." To protect the online contributors from any possible harm, the data were anonymized by replacing the usernames with pseudonyms, by making slight alterations to the dates of the comments directly cited, and by removing the names of specific items or medications. Even though more substantial changes to the content of each of these comments would have further diminished the chances of re-identification, a decision was made against this approach. This decision was informed by the consideration that only the authors of the online contributions are entitled to operate changes to them. Furthermore, even slight modifications to their content may have led to shifts in meaning and possible interpretations, which was deemed particularly undesirable, given that this book's aim is to show how online contributors diagnosed with bipolar disorder engage in knowledge practices. All quotes are, therefore, provided verbatim. Given their public standing, an exception to anonymization was made in the case of the two bloggers discussed in Chap. 5. Both bloggers were contacted and they are referred to in this book according to their own indication.

Outline of the Remaining Chapters

Chapter 2 traces the development of expertise about mental health from the early days of the asylum to the hopes and anxieties that are currently generated by the (upcoming) use of digital and AI-based technologies in the provision of mental healthcare. Based on a review of relevant historical and sociological works, it highlights the trajectory that expertise about mental health has undergone from the focus on heredity in the nineteenth century to the more recent embrace of genetics. In so doing, it engages with the jurisdictional struggles that emerged between psychiatry, psychology, and other disciplines, with the development of self-help and support groups in the US and France and with the precarious state that characterizes the provision of mental healthcare in both countries these days. By building an arch between the past and future of expertise about mental healthcare, this chapter provides rich contextual information which is important to better understand the online practices discussed in the remainder of the book and the similarities and differences among French and American contributors that will be described.

Chapter 3 describes how expertise about bipolar disorder is performed by *The National Institute of Mental Health* (NIMH) in the US and *La Haute Autorité de Santé* (HAS) in France. The analysis helps us understand how expertise is performed online by influential stakeholders, which possess substantial resources and have numerous options to choose from in terms of digital practices. The information NIMH and HAS put forward online about bipolar disorder was analyzed by combining insights from Latour (1987) and media studies with a dramaturgical perspective (Goffman, 1959/1990). This approach allowed for a better understanding of the material and epistemic relations that these institutions had to develop and manage online to successfully perform expertise. I argue that both stakeholders are rather reluctant Internet users, who perform expertise in a highly conservative fashion, which in turn allows them to articulate the knowledge currently available on this condition as stable and precise. While both institutions use similar performative techniques, they adapt them to subtly redefine bipolar disorder in ways which seem better aligned to the priorities characterizing their national health system and their institutional prerogatives and goals.

Chapter 4 traces how authoritative medical knowledge, such as that described above, permeates different areas of society, and becomes amenable to multiple usages and interpretations. It explores the Internet's democratizing potential by considering how people diagnosed with bipolar disorder re-appropriate medical perspectives and combine them with personal insights to contribute to the development of new knowledge through dynamic and even fleeting online exchanges on blogs and fora. This chapter is based on two types of sources: articles published by scientists in medical journals and data collected from blogs and fora, where people diagnosed shared their treatment experiences. I use de Certeau's theory (1988) of creative tactics in everyday life to analyze the online data, as it allows to move beyond domination and resistance as characterizing the main positions people diagnosed can develop in relation to dominant forms of knowledge, and to identify more subtle ways through which they can make their agency manifest. The analysis thus indicates that through their online interactions, people diagnosed move beyond the performance of lay expertise and collectively generate what I call "digitally informed hypotheses" in areas where the currently available medical knowledge on the effects and side effects of medications is insufficient. In so doing, the Internet affords individuals diagnosed a voice, yet one which can have a broad epistemic impact only when heard and taken seriously by researchers.

Chapter 5 shows that the Internet does not always favor the powerful, but this still does not mean that it has a democratizing effect. It traces the online activities of two bloggers diagnosed with bipolar disorder using the concept of interactional expertise developed by Collins and Evans (2002). This chapter argues that by combining medical knowledge with their situated experiences, and by utilizing the affordances of blogs, these bloggers have become a new type of stakeholder, what I call "online expert mediators." This chapter makes a theoretical contribution, as the notion of interactional expertise is extended by taking into consideration the role of the medium through which interactional expertise is displayed and by showing that its bi-directional character is more substantial than Collins and Evans initially envisaged. The analysis further indicates that the high standing of online expert mediators is not the result of a subversive use of the Internet, but of a dynamic alliance with "traditional" experts and of a strong media presence.

Chapter 6 builds upon recent calls made by medical sociologists and STS scholars to focus on the relational character of illness, thereby exploring the Internet's potential for solidarity. It shows that mental health-related online exchanges enable people diagnosed with bipolar disorder to perform solidarity. This has important epistemic consequences, because online solidaristic practices allow individuals both to perform lay expertise and to contribute to its collective development, as new knowledge is distilled from the personal experiences and insights that are brought together. Such activities are underpinned by affective labor, which facilitates the emergence of digital biocommunities and the development of lay expertise. Based on Prainsack and Buyx (2017)'s concept of solidarity and Gershon's (2010) notion of idioms of practice, the notion of digital biocommunities denotes a new type of subgroup, developed not only upon a common diagnosis, life circumstances, experiences, perspectives, and values, but also on similar engagements with the technologies of fora. By putting forward this concept, I highlight that despite an increased focus on individualization in mental healthcare, people diagnosed experience their condition in relational terms, even in regard to lived, embodied experiences.

Chapter 7 brings together the main findings and conclusions that have emerged from the study of the online performance of expertise about bipolar disorder described in this book. By building upon the theoretical perspectives discussed in this introductory chapter and by combining them with insights acquired from the empirical chapters, a new perspective on expertise was put forward. This new approach conceives of expertise as a practical and collective achievement realized through coordination and affective labor among stakeholders who occupy multiple and shifting positions within a complex ecosystem. This approach seeks to do justice to the important ways in which cultural and institutional factors shape expertise, while acknowledging the agency and complex identities of relevant stakeholders, who can be in turn or at the same time individuals diagnosed with a condition, professionals, scientific contributors, and information mediators. I discuss the significance of the main findings by considering them within the context of broader transformations that digital technologies have contributed to in processes of knowledge production, circulation, and evaluation, and which were already touched upon in Chap. 2. I argue that we need to move beyond rather simplistic approaches which see the Internet either as a quick technological fix or a postmodern version of Pandora's box.

References

Akrich, M. (2010). From Communities of Practice to Epistemic Communities: Health Mobilizations on the Internet. *Sociological Research Online, 15*(2), 10. Available at: http://www.socresonline.org.uk/15/2/10.html

Alda, M., Grof, P., Rouleau, G., Turecki, G., & Young, T. (2005). Investigating Responders to Lithium Prophylaxis as a Strategy for Mapping Susceptibility Genes for Bipolar Disorder. *Progress in Neuro-Psychopharmacology and Biological Psychiatry, 29*(6), 1038–1045.

American Psychiatric Association. (2013). Diagnostic and Statistical Manual of Mental Disorders, fifth edition (DSM-5).

Angst, J., & Marneros, A. (2001). Bipolarity from Ancient to Modern Times: Conception, Birth and Rebirth. *Journal of Affective Disorders, 67*, 3–19.

Angst, J., & Sellaro, R. (2000). Historical Perspectives and Natural History of Bipolar Disorder. *Biological Psychiatry, 48*, 445–457.

Ardichvili, A., Maurer, M., Wei, L., Wentling, T., & Stuedemann, R. (2006). Cultural Influences on Knowledge Sharing Through Online Communities of Practice. *Journal of Knowledge Management, 10*(1), 94–107.

Barad, K. (2003). Posthumanist Performativity: Toward an Understanding of How Matter Comes to Matter. *Signs, 28*(3), 801–831.

Bar-Ilan, J., Mat-Hassan, M., & Levene, M. (2006). Methods for Comparing Rankings of Search Engine Results. *Computer Networks, 50*, 1448–1463.

Barnes, B. (1974). *Scientific Knowledge and Sociological Theory*. Routledge & Kegan Paul.

Bijker, W. (1995). *Of Bicycles, Bakelites, and Bulbs: Toward a Theory of the Sociotechnical Change*. The MIT Press.

Bishop, S. (2018). Anxiety, Panic and Self-Optimization: Inequalities and the YouTube Algorithm. *Convergence, 24*(1), 69–84.

Bloor, D. (1976). *Knowledge and Social Imagery*. Routledge & Kegan Paul.

British Psychological Society (BPS). (2013). *Ethics Guidelines for Internet-Mediated Research*. British Psychological Society.

Brown, B., & Baker, S. (2012). *Responsible Citizens. Individuals, Health and Policy under Neoliberalism*. Anthem Press.

Carron-Arthur, B., Reynolds, J., Bennett, K., Bennett, A., Cunningham, J., & Griffiths, K. (2016). Community Structure of a Mental Health Internet Support Group: Modularity in User Thread Participation. *JMIR Mental Health, 3*(2), e20.

Collins, H., & Evans, R. (2002). The Third Wave of Science Studies. Studies of Expertise and Experience. *Social Studies of Science, 32*(2), 235–296.

Collins, H., & Evans, R. (2007). *Re-thinking Expertise*. The University of Chicago Press.

Collins, H., Evans, R., & Weinel, M. (2017). Interactional Expertise. In U. Felt, R. Fouché, C. Miller, & L. Smith-Doerr (Eds.), *The Handbook of Science and Technology Studies* (4th ed., pp. 765–792). The MIT Press.

Cruceanu, C., Alda, M., & Turecki, G. (2009). Lithium: A Key to the Genetics of Bipolar Disorder. *Genome Medicine, 1*(8), 79.

Davis, J., & Chouinard, J. (2016). Theorizing Affordances: From Request to Refuse. *Bulletin of Science, Technology & Society, 36*(4), 241–248.

de Certeau, M. (1988). *The Practice of Everyday Life*. University of California Press.

Dedding, C., van Doorn, R., Winker, L., & Reis, R. (2011). How Will e-health Affect Patient Participation in the Clinic? A review of e-health Studies and the Current Evidence for Changes in the Relationship between Medical Professionals and Patients. *Social Science & Medicine, 72*(1), 49–53.

Dehue, T. (2008). *De Depressie-Epidemie*. Augustus.

Dreyfus, H., & Dreyfus, S. (1986). *Mind Over Machine: The Power of Human Intuition and Expertise in the Era of the Computer*. Free Press.

Drucker, J. (2011). Humanities Approaches to Interface Theory. *Culture Machine, 12*. Available at: http://www.culturemachine.net/index.php/cm/article/view/434/462

Edwards, A. (2010). *Being an Expert Professional Practitioner. The Relational Turn in Expertise*. Springer.

Engeström, Y. (2018). *Expertise in Transition. Expansive Learning in Medical Work*. Cambridge University Press.

Esposito, L., & Perez, F. (2014). Neoliberalism and the Commodification of Mental Health. *Humanity & Society, 38*(4), 414–442.

Evetts, J., Mieg, H., & Felt, U. (2006). Professionalization, Scientific Expertise and Elitism: A Sociological Perspective. In K. Ericsson, N. Charness, P. Feltovich, & R. Hoffman (Eds.), *The Cambridge Handbook of Expertise and Expert Performance* (pp. 105–123). Cambridge University Press.

Eyal, G. (2013). For a Sociology of Expertise: The Social Origins of the Autism Epidemic. *American Journal of Sociology, 118*(4), 863–907.

Eyal, G., & Hart, B. (2010). How Parents of Autistic Children Became "Experts on Their Own Children": Notes Towards a Sociology of Expertise. *Annual Conference of the Berkeley Journal of Sociology, 54*, 1–38. Available at https://works.bepress.com/gil_eyal/1/

Eyal, G., Hart, B., Onculer, E., Oren, N., & Rossi, N. (2010). *The Autism Matrix: The Social Origins of the Autism Epidemic*. Polity Press.

Eysenbach, G., Powell, J., Englesakis, M., Rizo, C., & Stern, A. (2004). Health Related Virtual Communities and Electronic Support Groups: Systematic

Review of The Effects of Online Peer to Peer Interactions. *British Medical Journal, 328*(7449), 1166–1170.

Featherstone, M., Lash, S., & Robertson, R. (Eds.). (1995). *Global Modernities*. Sage Publications.

Foucault, M. (1972/2010). *History of Madness*. Routledge. Translated by Jonathan Murphy and Jean Khalfa.

Fox, N., Ward, K., & O'Rourke, A. (2005). The "Expert Patient": Empowerment or Medical Dominance? The Case of Weight Loss, Pharmaceutical Drugs and the Internet. *Social Science & Medicine, 69*, 1299–1309.

Fuller, S. (2017). The Post-Truth about Philosophy and Rhetoric. *Philosophy & Rhetoric, 50*(4), 473–482.

Gershon, I. (2010). *The Breakup 2.0. Disconnecting over New Media*. Cornell University Press. E-book.

Goffman, E. (1959/1990). *The Presentation of Self in Everyday Life* (8th ed.). Penguin.Mol.

Grande, I., Berk, M., Birmaher, B., & Vieta, E. (2016). Bipolar Disorder. *The Lancet, 387*(10027), 1561–1572.

Hacking, I. (1995). *Rewriting the Soul: Multiple Personality and the Sciences of Memory*. Princeton University Press.

Hacking, I. (1999). *The Social Construction of What?* Harvard University Press.

Hafermalz, E., Riemer, K., & Boell, S. (2016). Enactment of Performance? A Non-dualist Reading of Goffman. In L. Introna, D. Kavanagh, S. Kelly, W. Orlikowski, & S. Scott (Eds.), *Beyond Interpretivism? New Encounters with Technology and Organization* (pp. 167–181). Springer.

Hardey, M. (1999). Doctor in the House: The Internet as A Source of Lay Health Knowledge and the Challenge to Expertise. *Sociology of Health & Illness, 21*, 820–835.

Harding, S. (Ed.). (2004). *The Feminist Standpoint Theory Reader. Intellectual and Political Controversies*. Routledge.

Hargittai, E. (2007). The Social, Political, Economic and Cultural Dimensions of Search Engines: An Introduction. *Journal of Computer-Mediated Communication, 12*(3), 769–777.

Healy, D. (2008). *Mania: A Short History of Bipolar Disorder*. John Hopkins University Press.

Herring, S. (2012). Discourse in Web 2.0.: Familiar, Reconfigured, and Emergent. In D. Tannen & A. Tester (Eds.), *Georgetown University Round Table on Languages and Linguistics 2011: Discourse 2.0.: Language and new media* (pp. 1–29). Georgetown University Press.

Hidaka, B. (2012). Depression as a Disease of Modernity: Explanations for Increasing Prevalence. *Journal of Affective Disorders, 140*, 205–214.

Höchstötter, N., & Lewandowski, D. (2009). What Users See — Structures in Search Engine Results Pages. *Information Sciences, 179*, 1796–1812.

Hogle, L. (2016). Data-intensive Resourcing in Healthcare. *BioSocieties, 11*(3), 372–393.

Horwitz, A., & Wakefield, J. (2007). *The Loss of Sadness. How Psychiatry Transformed Normal Sorrow into Depressive Disorder*. Oxford University Press.

Hu, Y., & Sundar, S. (2010). Effects of Online Health Sources on Credibility and Behavioral Intentions. *Communication Research, 31*(1), 105–132.

Illich, I. (1977). *Disabling Professions*. Marion Boyars.

Jasanoff, S. (2003). Breaking the Waves in Science Studies: Comment on H.M. Collins and Robert Evans, 'The Third Wave of Science Studies'. *Social Studies of Science, 33*(3), 389–400.

Jasanoff, S. (Ed.). (2004). *States of Knowledge. The Co-Production of Science and Social Order*. Routledge.

Kitcher, P. (2011). *Science in a Democratic Society*. Prometheus Books.

Kivits, J. (2009). Everyday Health and the Internet: A Mediated Health Perspective on Health Information Seeking. *Sociology of Health and Illness, 31*(5), 673–687.

Kleinman, A. (1988). *Rethinking Psychiatry from Cultural Category to Personal Experience*. The Free Press.

Koppl, R. (2010). The Social Construction of Expertise. *Society, 47*(3), 220–226.

Kotzee, B. (2014). Differentiating Forms of Professional Expertise. In M. Young & J. Muller (Eds.), *Knowledge, Expertise and the Professions* (pp. 61–76). Routledge.

Kotzee, B., & Smit, J. (2017). Two Social Dimensions of Expertise. *Journal of Philosophy of Education, 51*(3), 640–654.

Lakoff, A. (2005). *Pharmaceutical Reason: Knowledge and Value in Global Psychiatry*. Cambridge University Press.

Latour, B. (1987). *Science in Action. How to Follow Scientists and Engineers Through Society*. Harvard University Press.

Lupton, D. (2018). *Digital Health*. Routledge.

Lynch, D. (2017). STS, Symmetry and Post-Truth. *Social Studies of Science, 47*(4), 593–599.

MacQueen, G., Young, L., & Joffe, R. (2001). A Review of the Psychosocial Outcomes in Patients with Bipolar Disorder. *Acta Psychiatrica Scandinavica, 103*(3), 163–170.

Markham, A. (2016). Method as Ethic, Ethic as Method. *Journal of Information Ethics, 15*(2), 37–55.

Martin, E. (2009). *Bipolar Expeditions. Mania and Depression in American Culture* (2nd ed.). Princeton University Press.

McNeil, M. (1998). Gender, Expertise and Feminism. In R. Williams, W. Faulkner, & J. Fleck (Eds.), *Exploring Expertise: Issues and Perspectives* (pp. 55–79). Macmillan Press.

Metzl, J. (2009). *The Protest Psychosis. How Schizophrenia Became a Black Disease.* Beacon Press.

Miller, D., & Slater, D. (2000). *The Internet. An Ethnographic Approach.* Berg.

Mitchell, R., & Waldby, C. (2010). National Biobanks: Clinical Labor, Risk Production, and the Creation of Biovalue. *Science, Technology & Human Values, 35*(3), 330–355.

Mol, A. (2002). *The Body Multiple: Ontology in Medical Practice.* Duke University Press.

Naslund, J., Aschbrenner, K., Marsch, L., & Bartels, S. (2016). The Future of Mental Health Care: Peer-To-Peer Support and Social Media. *Epidemiology and Psychiatric Sciences, 25*(2), 113–122.

National Conference of State Legislatures. (2018, February 20). Value-Based Insurance Design. Retrieved from http://www.ncsl.org/research/health/value-based-insurance-design.aspx. Accessed on December 30, 2018.

Neff, G. (2013). Why Big Data Won't Cure Us. *Big Data, 1*, 117–123. PMID:25161827.

Nettleton, S., & Burrows, R. (2003). E-Scaped Medicine? Information, Reflexivity, and Health. *Critical Social Policy, 23*(2), 165–185.

Nielsen, K., & Langstrup, H. (2018). Tactics of Material Participation: How Patients Shape Their Engagement through E-health. *Social Studies of Science, 48*(2), 259–282.

Orgad, S. (2005). The Transformative Potential of Online Communication. *Feminist Media Studies 5*(2), 141–161.

Pasquinelli, M. (2009). Google's PageRank Algorithm: A Diagram of the Cognitive Capitalism and the Rentier of the Common Intellect. In K. Becker & F. Stalder (Eds.), *Deep Search: The Politics of Search Beyond Google* (pp. 152–162). Transaction Publishers.

Poster, M. (2001). *What's The Matter with The Internet?* University of Minnesota Press.

Prainsack, B. (2011). Voting with Their Mice: Personal Genome Testing and the "Participatory Turn" in Disease Research. *Accountability in Research, 18*(3), 132–147.

Prainsack, B. (2018). The "We" in the "Me": Solidarity and Health Care in the Era of Personalized Medicine. *Science, Technology, & Human Values, 43*(1), 21–44.

Prainsack, B., & Buyx, A. (2017). *Solidarity in Biomedicine and Beyond.* Cambridge University Press.

Radder, H. (2018, April 16). Post-Truth en de Vraag Wat Goede Wetenschap Is. *Science Guide.* Retrieved April 20, 2018, from https://www.scienceguide. nl/2018/04/de-vraag-wat-is-goede-wetenschap-blijft-relevant/

Richmond, K. (2017, August 29). Towards a Feminist Theory of Expertise. *The Postgraduate Gender Research Network of Scotland.* Retrieved May 21, 2018, from https://pgrnscotland.wordpress.com/2017/08/29/towards-a-feminist-theory-of-expertise/

Rose, N. (1992). Engineering the Human Soul: Analyzing Psychological Expertise. *Science in Context, 5*(2), 351–369.

Rose, N. (2018). *Our Psychiatric Futures.* Polity.

Saks, M. (2012). Defining a Profession. *Professions and Professionalism, 2*(11), 1–10.

Scott, S. (2006). The Medicalisation of Shyness: From Social Misfits to Social Fitness. *Sociology of Health & Illness, 28*(2), 133–153.

Selinger, E., & Crease, R. (2006). Dreyfus on Expertise. The Limits of Phenomenological Analysis. In E. Selinger & R. Crease (Eds.), *The Philosophy of Expertise.* Columbia University Press.

Shapin S, Schaffer S (1985/2011). *Leviathan and the Air-Pump. Hobbes, Boyle, and the Experimental Life.* 2nd ed. Princeton: Princeton University Press.

Sharon, T. (2016). The Googlization of Health Research: From Disruptive Innovation to Disruptive Ethics. *Personalized Medicine, 13*(6), 563–574.

Sismondo, S. (2017). Post-Truth? *Social Studies of Science, 47*(1), 3–6.

Stommel, W., & Lamerichs, J. (2014). Interaction in Online Support Groups. Advice and Beyond. In H. Hamilton & W. Chou (Eds.), *The Routledge Handbook of Language and Health Communication* (pp. 198–211). Routledge.

Susskind, R., & Susskind, D. (2015). *The Future of the Professions. How Technology Will Transform the Work of Human Experts.* Oxford University Press.

Terranova, T. (2000). Free Labor: Producing Culture for the Digital Economy. *Social Text 63, 18*(2), 33–58.

Topol, E. (2015). *The Patient Will See You Now. The Future of Medicine Is in Your Hands.* Basic Books.

Tutton, R., & Prainsack, B. (2011). Enterprising or Altruistic Selves? Making Up Research Subjects in Genetics Research. *Sociology of Health & Illness, 33*(7), 1081–1095.

Vaugrente, C. (2018, March 29). Troubles Bipolaires: Les Différences Femmes/ Hommes. Retrieved from https://www.e-sante.fr/troubles-bipolaires-les-differences-femmeshommes/actualite/615617. Accessed on April 15, 2018.

Versteeg, W., & Te Molder, H. (2018). "You Must Know What You Mean When You Say That": The Morality of Knowledge Claims about ADHD in Radio Phone-Ins. *Sociology of Health & Illness, 40*(4), 1–17.

Waldby, C., & Cooper, M. (2008). The Biopolitics of Reproduction. *Australian Feminist Studies, 23*(55), 57–73.

Whiteford, A., Degenhardt, L., Rehm, J., Baxter, A., Ferrari, A., Erskine, H., Charlson, F., Norman, R., Flaxman, A., Johns, N., Burstein, R., Murray, C., & Vos, T. (2013). Global Burden of Disease Attributable to Mental and Substance Use Disorders: Findings from the Global Burden of Disease Study 2010. *The Lancet, 382*(9904), 1575–1586.

Williams, R., Faulkner, W., & Fleck, J. (Eds.). (1998). *Exploring Expertise. Issues and Perspectives.* Macmillan Press.

World Health Organization. (WHO). (2010). International Statistical Classification of Diseases and Related Health Problems, 10th Revision (ICD-10). World Health Organization.

Wyatt, S., Harris, A., Adams, S., & Kelly, S. (2013). Illness Online: Self-Reported Data and Questions of Trust in Medical and Social Research. *Theory, Culture & Society, 30*(4), 131–150.

Wyatt, S., Harris, A., & Kelly, S. (2016). Controversy Goes Online: Schizophrenia Genetics on Wikipedia. *Science & Technology Studies, 29*(1), 13–29.

Young, M., & Muller, J. (Eds.). (2014). *Knowledge, Expertise and the Professions.* Routledge.

Ziebland, S., & Wyke, S. (2012). Health and Illness in a Connected World: How Might Sharing Experiences on the Internet Affect People's Health? *The Milbank Quarterly, 90*(2), 219–249.

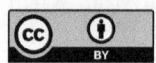

2

Epistemic Inroads from the Asylum to Digital Psychiatry

Expertise about mental health has been marked since its early days by an important set of challenges, which it has not yet managed to fully overcome. Psychiatry's recognition as a medical specialty in its own right, the scientific character of its methods, the effectiveness of its therapeutic interventions, its political functions, and the struggle between care and cure have marked its history (Rose, 2018). Important have also been the various jurisdictional struggles in which psychiatry has been embroiled, as authority over various areas of mental health has been claimed by different disciplines, which have developed or become more influential over the years due to the availability of new types of tools and knowledge. These aspects are important in view of the new conceptualization of expertise that I put forward, where epistemic practices are shaped by the ecosystem within which they develop, which frames their conditions of possibility. Based on this understanding, expertise about bipolar disorder online emerges at the confluence of specific historical trajectories that have shaped how and what has been studied in relation to mental health conditions, of current needs and circumstances in this healthcare sector, and of expectations about the future. To better understand the online practices that this book focuses on, this chapter draws an arch, stretching

© The Author(s) 2023
C. Egher, *Digital Healthcare and Expertise*, Health, Technology and Society,
https://doi.org/10.1007/978-981-16-9178-2_2

from the establishment of asylums at the beginning of the nineteenth century to the current provision of mental healthcare in the US and France and the future visions animating it. Such a broad longitudinal perspective means that while important elements will be highlighted, many complex debates will be simplified and a series of aspects that are not directly relevant for the argument made in this book will be overlooked. These shortcomings are mitigated, however, by the fact that the understanding of the online practices discussed in the following chapters will be enriched through the historical insights and future hopes and fears about the digitalization of mental healthcare (Pickersgill, 2019) described here. This will allow us to better appreciate the novelty but also the continuity that underscores them.

Historical Overview of the Development of Expertise About Mental Health

Significant for the development of expertise about mental health are the changes that took place at the end of the eighteenth century, when the realization that community care for the "insane" often involved abusive approaches prompted many to advocate for the necessity of "moral treatments" and the establishment of asylums as the means to achieve this. Since it was largely thought that "madness" was triggered and/or aggravated by the circumstances one found oneself in, asylums were envisioned as tranquil, orderly places, where one could recover from the humdrum of modernity and industrialization. Thus, in the early days, at least, the establishment of asylums was animated by humanistic tendencies, by the desire to cure those afflicted by "madness" and to provide them and their families with support and solace. From this point of view, the asylum system could be understood as a precursor and important influence on the development of the welfare state, as Porter (2018) convincingly argued. Its spread was encouraged in France by the 1838 law which required mental health facilities to be established in each département, and similar legislation was soon passed also in the US. Throughout the nineteenth century and beyond, mental healthcare continued to be provided in various ways, within the community and across other institutions, such as university hospitals and private clinics (Rose, 2018). Where one received mental healthcare depended not only on the facilities that were available in one's region, but also on one's socioeconomic status. In France, asylums were funded by the state, which helped inform a greater degree of centralization and standardization of practices, even though important differences were recorded between departments depending on the availability of such facilities. In the US, their funding depended on legislation and the preferred policies and approaches at the level of the individual states, which led to greater variability and disparities. As we shall see in the next chapter, such differences made a durable mark upon the organization of the mental healthcare systems in these two countries and can also be noted these days.

The establishment of asylums played an important role in the development of "mental medicine" as it made it possible for alienists, the doctors treating the "mad," to study the behaviors of a great number of patients and to engage in various experiments. At the time, mental healthcare was provided based on the symptoms patients experienced and consisted of a combination of scientific and behavioral measures, which varied in duration, harshness, and intensity. Mental health conditions were distinguished based on groups of symptoms and they were thought to be brought about by physical, moral causes, or a combination of both. Distinctions were made between predisposing and effective causes, as it was thought that whereas one may have been susceptible to develop mental health issues due to bodily factors, a triggering event was needed to set such processes into motion. Such events were often of a moral nature, as can be noted by the numerous causes for mental illness that were circulated at the time, ranging from revolutionary excess and participation in political events, to sedentary occupations, and a low level of instruction (Porter, 2018).

This understanding of causes greatly shaped how mental health conditions were studied as well as how they were intervened upon. Alienists initially combined clinical and laboratory expertise, as they sought to locate these conditions within the body, and apart from the various examinations on asylum residents, they also engaged in postmortem investigations, focusing primarily on the brain. Yet, by the second decade of the nineteenth century, the lack of any reliable indication that markers of "madness" could be indisputably identified within pathological autonomy "were drawing the profession into crisis" (Arribas-Ayllon et al., 2019: 28). This prompted the alienists to focus on heredity, for which they had shown little interest prior to 1812, as a fundamental cause (Arribas-Ayllon et al., 2019; Foucault, 1972/2010). They understood heredity as a predisposing cause, which could trigger mental health conditions in combination with what were thought at the time as morally reprehensible behaviors, such as the consumption of alcohol, masturbation, and overwork. The study of heredity was accompanied by the development of new approaches and techniques, as it broadened the focus from the individuals afflicted by mental health issues to their families and made new types of data necessary, which could be acquired through detailed questioning, family history searches, and the development of family pedigrees. Even though the alienists enthusiastically engaged in the collection of vast amounts of data, the latter were not equally available across institutions, nor were they systematically collected from the very beginning. Substantial efforts were therefore dedicated to improve the quality of the data collected and to standardize the data collection methods, so as to facilitate comparisons and to enhance the scientific character of the insights acquired. An important landmark in this sense was Esquirol's use of the statistic table as a means to organize mental health cases in France, practice which became popular among many alienists, who soon improved on this technology in order to better determine correlations (Porter, 2018).

Psychiatric expertise thus came to rely on a combination of clinical and statistical knowledge, and the latter informed its development as a partially international enterprise. Knowledge was intensely exchanged among alienists through professional tours in the US and Europe, at international meetings organized by the numerous professional associations that were being established, and through the eager publication of their statistics in the specialty journals that were founded in considerable number from the 1840s onward (Porter, 2018). There were, however, also important differences among countries concerning the role ascribed to statistical knowledge in relation to psychiatric expertise and to what were considered the best means to study the impact of heredity on mental health. Thus, whether or not the deployment of statistical methods was an indication of scientific rather than merely administrative or bureaucratic expertise was the object of heated debates in France, where many mental healthcare professionals reproached their statistically bent colleagues for having a simplistic understanding of heredity and mental illness. Under their influence, the dominant understanding of "insane heredity" in France became that of a process of physical and mental decay where the environment played a complex role, and "insane heredity" continued to be studied through cases. This marks an important difference between the US and other European countries, such as Germany, where expertise about the heredity of mental health conditions was successfully claimed by statisticians and geneticists (Porter, 2018).

Despite the more standardized data collection and statistical methods used, the mechanisms through which heredity affected mental and bodily processes continued to remain unclear. The alienists managed, however, to successfully mobilize this uncertainty to position mental health as an important social issue, which required not only treatment, but also urgent social reforms focusing on prevention at the national level. In France, this process was facilitated by political developments, as medical practitioners came to play an important role in public health due to the Napoleonic reforms. As heredity's influence on the development of mental illness was thought to be rather grim, the alienists warned that it led to degeneration through its cumulative effects across multiple generations. Hereditary mental defects thus became a national concern, as they could impede a country's progress and competitiveness, and their management required a combination of scientific and moral approaches. The same ethos was exuded in the US by many asylum supporters, who argued in favor of a greater provision of funds for these institutions and for important social measures as an adequate response. In this context, the alienists successfully positioned the moral expertise they claimed to be endowed with as highly relevant, and came to "moralize the masses" (Arribas-Ayllon et al., 2019:30) by directing nation-wide efforts to eliminate the moral behaviors they found problematic. Through their work, from the 1840s onward, both in France and in the US, the population censuses started to collect data through which the spread of mental health conditions and the role of heredity in such processes were hoped to be determined at the level of the nation.

Such data collection processes went hand in hand with attempts to standardize diagnoses, yet mental health conditions proved difficult to classify. Initially, alienists such as Pinel sought to distinguish between mental health conditions based on their etiology, that is, on their causes and origins, but the failure to identify specific physical causes brought such an approach under strain. As asylums made possible the observation of the pattern of symptoms experienced by an individual over a period of time, at the end of the nineteenth century, the German psychiatrist Emil Kraepelin advanced the idea of establishing diagnoses based on prognosis rather than etiology through the collection of detailed histories of the course of illness. Kraepelin put forward a new nosology, where he identified 13 major groups of mental health conditions. Relevant here is the division of psychotic illnesses into "manic-depressive psychosis" and "dementia praecox," known these days as schizophrenia, which he introduced based on the presence or absence of mood changes and by focusing on their outcome. Whereas the latter was understood to lead to cognitive and clinical decline, the former allowed for a less pessimistic perspective (Healy, 2008), although the overall outlook remained grim. Kraepelin's approach was met with reserve in France, partly due to recent memories of the war between this country and Germany and to persistent political animosities. But it also stemmed from the fact that French psychiatrists did not share his negative perspective on the outcome of these conditions, with many of them arguing that Kraepelin's views had been skewed by his observations of asylum patients, who presented more aggravated forms of mental health conditions than those who could be seen by city doctors, for instance, in other medical institutions (Hochmann, 2017). In contrast, Kraepelin's focus on prognosis was initially enthusiastically received by Adolf Meyer, director of the New York State Psychiatric Institute and, through his influence, by many other American psychiatrists, who appreciated the return to a clinical focus in psychiatry. While Kraepelin's perspectives remained generally popular in the US, in the 1920s Meyer himself changed course, as he reproached the German psychiatrist for a too strong neurological focus, and he highlighted, instead, the role of the environment in the development and outcome of mental health conditions. Thus, in Meyer's view, mental health conditions were not so much the result of the cumulated effects of faulty genes but rather inadequate reactions to life circumstances that could be made sense of within the context of a patient's life (Healy, 2008; Hochmann, 2017; Rose, 2018) and that could be partially addressed and prevented through an adequate mental hygiene.

The search for diagnosis criteria based on etiology or prognosis marked a durable distinction among mental healthcare professionals of a different bent and was also reflected in their understanding of the role of genes in the development of mental health conditions. As the statistical data of populations came to be seen as a form of scientific capital at the beginning of the twentieth century (Arribas-Ayllon et al., 2019), it galvanized collaborations among alienists, statisticians, biologists, and so on and thereby challenged the separation between mental health expertise and "ordinary medicine" which had strongly persisted until then (Porter, 2018). Hopes of establishing mental health diagnoses based on etiology were revitalized by such collaborations through a renewed focus on the brain, on the one hand, and on the influence of genes, on the other. Thus, neurological and experimental approaches regained popularity among some mental healthcare professionals in the US, who thought the psychiatry of the asylums with its focus on clinical observations was outdated. For instance, the New York asylums purchased freezing microtomes for slicing brain samples, which they used for various investigations and preserved along with cards describing the behavioral profile of the person they were coming from, as even after the 1930s, some hoped to correlate characteristics of the preserved brain with the actions and behaviors of "insane" criminals. Also in France, a renewed focus on the neural and molecular mechanisms underlying specific symptoms could be noted, with neuropsychiatrists such as Clérambault arguing that delirious and hallucinatory states were the result of the irritation of nerve centers that could gradually engulf the entire cortex (Hochmann, 2017).

The role of genes in the development of mental health conditions acquired renewed attention, as important breakthroughs in the realm of statistics, such as Galton's probabilistic laws, allowed for mathematical relationships to be determined among generations in terms of hereditary transmission (Arribas-Ayllon et al., 2019). Further impetus was provided by the (re)discovery of the Mendelian ratios and the attempts to apply them in the study of the development of mental health conditions.

Noteworthy in this sense are the activities of the American researchers Davenport, Goddard, and Rosanoff, who tried to persuade their European counterparts that insanity could be explained as single-factor Mendelian traits, that is, that discrete genetic units could be linked with specific mental health conditions, such as manic-depressive illness, as bipolar disorder was largely known at the time. Heated debates emerged about the role of genes between such Mendelian supporters, many of whom were neuropsychiatrists, who considered different mental health conditions to be determined by specific groups of rare genes, and biometricians and clinical psychiatrists who argued that mental health conditions were triggered through the concerted influence of rare variants and multiple genes of small effects. The biometricians and statisticians found issue with the quality of the data and of the calculations upon which those in favor of Mendelism based their claims, whereas the psychiatrists found a clinical approach based on the long-term observation of the patient and the development of the disease more reliable and useful (Arribas-Ayllon et al., 2019; Porter, 2018).

By the end of the nineteenth century, the failure of the asylums had become obvious in both the US and France, as the number of people diagnosed with mental health conditions was on the rise, while the effectiveness of the treatments used remained limited. Different types of mental healthcare professionals embraced therefore hereditarianism. Some did this because the broader correlations heredity allowed for between physical and moral causes enabled them to claim expertise on various social matters (Arribas-Ayllon et al., 2019; Porter, 2018). Others became involved in social reforms and other political decisions pertaining to the management of populations, as it provided them with access to the resources and influence needed to continue their neurological and genetic studies (Porter, 2018). Heredity thus became entwined with themes of family and racial hygiene, as the research activities pursued by Davenport and his supporters in the US illustrate. Furthermore, next to warning against certain behaviors, the alienists came to give advice on reproductive practices. Psychiatry was thus from its early days a political science (Rose, 2018), which not only exerted negative power through prohibitions and forced commitment into asylums, but also positive power, as it encouraged the "healthy" population to "breed." Nevertheless, it is important to bear in mind that, for at least the first half of the twentieth century, the trajectories of psychiatric genetics and neuropsychiatry were marked by the suffering, exclusion, and extermination brought about by mental healthcare professionals involved in the eugenics movement or collaborating with authoritarian political regimes. This, however, did not put an end to the claims of mental healthcare professionals to moral expertise, as they remain important to our present time, as we will now see, as we turn our focus to Freud and psychoanalysis.

While psychiatrists sought to determine the causes of mental health conditions by focusing on genes or on the brain, their jurisdiction over the field of mental health came to be disputed at the end of the nineteenth century by dynamic psychologists, who introduced a different perspective by focusing on trauma and its impact on individual development. Having studied in France, Freud was critical of the wide role ascribed there to heredity and degeneration in relation to mental health conditions (Hochmann, 2017). He argued, instead, in favor of a focus on the individual and its development, which Freud thought to be importantly shaped by circumstances unfolding in the private sphere (Hochmann, 2017; Illlouz, 2008). In France, the uptake of psychoanalysis was very slow and Freud's views remained largely unpopular until the 1960s (Turkle, 1981). The first French psychoanalytic association was founded only in 1926, more than a decade after its American counterpart, and this new approach to mental healthcare was generally disregarded by reputed French mental healthcare professionals as well as by vast numbers of the population, who considered it a new form of bourgeois self-indulgence (Turkle, 1981). In the US, however, psychoanalysis enjoyed tremendous popularity from its very beginning, at the confluence of three main factors: the ongoing jurisdictional struggles among medical professionals and representatives of the clergy about the provision of mental healthcare; the popularity of spiritual approaches and interventions focusing on the mind; and the ambivalence of Freud's theories which allowed various stakeholders to adopt them in the pursuit of distinct goals (Illlouz, 2008).

The support of the American medical elites for psychoanalysis ensured its development as a medical specialty in its own right and its embedding within influential institutions. Already in the second decade of the twentieth century, numerous professional psychoanalytic societies were formed, the first American psychoanalytic journals, *The Psychoanalytic Review* and *The Psychoanalytic Quarterly*, were published, and uniform professional criteria were developed in a bid to heighten its authority and legitimacy. Furthermore, in 1927, the American Psychoanalytic Society decided that only medical doctors were allowed to train and practice as psychoanalysts (Illlouz, 2008), which enhanced its "domestication" (Turkle, 1981). The treatment of bipolar disorder in the US, over which psychiatrists had dominated, thus also came under the purview of psychoanalysts, who were importantly influenced by the works of Abraham, one of Freud's supporters and collaborators on *On Murder, Mourning and Melancholia* (1917/2005). Abraham focused on the study of psychoses and considered bipolar disorder to be the result of libidinal fixations that ensued as an infant's sexual development was frustrated. In his view, bipolar disorder thus constituted a reenactment of past conflicts informed by the ambivalence of the loved object. Abraham developed various methods through which psychoanalytic approaches could be employed as therapeutic practices for bipolar disorder and exerted a strong influence on Lewin's thinking, an important member of the New York Psychoanalytic Society. Under the influence of Erikson and Maslow, the ultimate goal of therapy came to be self-realization (Illlouz, 2008), which enabled psychologists to claim expertise over broad areas of social and private life, thus continuing the moral careers initiated by nineteenth-century alienists.

The publication of the first Diagnostic and Statistical Manual (DSM-I) in 1952 indicated that expertise about mental healthcare in the US was largely shaped at the time by psychoanalytic perspectives and by Meyer's psychobiological style of thought (Illlouz, 2008; Rose, 2018). The manual distinguished between mental health conditions that developed as a result of impaired brain functioning and psychiatric conditions, such as depression of phobia, which were thought to arise as the result of maladaptive behaviors. This latter group of conditions was seen as reactions to environmental circumstances rather than as full-fledged disease entities (Rose, 2018). This meant that an important aspect of therapeutic practice consisted of mental healthcare professionals' activities of interpretation of the symptoms exhibited by a person, which had to be made sense within the life story of the person diagnosed. This perspective

triggered, however, intense reactions from mental healthcare professionals who considered this a threat to the scientific character of psychiatric
diagnoses, leading to the removal of the term "reactions" from DSM-II
(1968) and to the pronounced biological and clinical focus at the heart of
DSM-III (Healy, 2008; Rose, 2018). Under the strong influence of a
group of psychiatrists at the Department of Psychiatry of the University
of Washington, the 1970s were marked by a "major epistemological and
ontological shift" (Rose, 2018:79) with the return to etiology in diagnosis, and the search for biological causes as underlying, even when partial,
causes of disease. Expertise about mental healthcare was thus hoped to
become more objective, as diagnoses were based upon observable symptoms, and, where applicable, upon laboratory tests, which were expected
to be understood in the same way by any mental healthcare professional
assessing them.

The 1980s were therefore marked by an acceleration of studies conducted to discover the neurological processes or the genetic factors underlying bipolar disorder and other related conditions. In psychiatric
genetics, family and twin studies were taken up again, whereas technological developments, such as recombinant DNA and advances in chro-
mosomal mapping, allowed for the construction of genetic linkage maps,
thereby briefly bringing back to life and popularity the idea of single
dominant genes the Mendelians had been so fond of (Arribas-Ayllon
et al., 2019). Several claims about the identification of genes for bipolar
disorder were made in the second part of the 1980s (Baron et al., 1987;
Egeland et al., 1987), but they failed to be replicated. Even though the
more advanced technologies developed in the aftermath of the Human
Genome Project in early 2000 resurrected hopes about a more thorough
understanding of the mechanisms through which genes were involved in
the development of mental health conditions such as bipolar disorder, the
results remained rather disappointing. Thus, at the entry into the new
millennium bipolar disorder was considered to be the result of complex
genetic traits, which "provide[d] theoretical coherence and respectability
to an otherwise ambivalent relationship between genetic and non-genetic
factors" (Arribas-Ayllon et al., 2019:75). Even though no biomarkers
could be used as reliable indicators of diagnoses even by the time the latest DSM-5 (2013) was published, the widespread use of digital

technologies and advances in AI have nourished hopes that before long a precision medicine psychiatry will be within reach. The efforts to develop medical knowledge and therapeutic approaches for mental health conditions sketched thus far were also accompanied by important activities focusing on the provision of care, whereby support and self-help groups played an important role, as I briefly highlight below.

Self-help and Support Groups

The history of psychiatry has been profoundly marked by its confrontation with a double "temptation"—the provision of therapeutic care and that of social assistance (Swain, 1988). Given this book's empirical focus on the activities of people diagnosed with bipolar disorder and since "the emergence of support groups should be understood as the other side of the cultural coin of institutionalized therapeutic language" (Illlouz, 2008:186), it is important to briefly consider the role self-help and social support groups have historically played. In France, such groups have started to develop in the aftermath of the Second World War. A noteworthy landmark in the development of support groups, which consisted of both medical professionals and people diagnosed, was the founding of the Croix Marine movement (*Fédération d'Aide à la Santé Mentale Croix Marine*). It was initiated by three psychiatrists—Pierre Doussinet, Alice Delaunay, and Elizabeth Jacob—in 1952, with the aim of providing protection and mutual psychological and social help to people diagnosed with mental health conditions. While over the following two decades the provision of ambulatory care launched this way developed further, changes in French legislation in the 1970s regarding the status and prerogatives of social and medico-social institutions led to a strict separation between the provision of medical care and social action.

Inspired by the 1968 protests, a number of psychiatrists together with people diagnosed with mental health conditions founded the *Groupe d'Information Asile* (GIA) in the early 1970s (Bernadet et al., 2002), to fight against repressive practices in psychiatry. The group has since developed a strong juridical orientation and claims to have played a major contribution in the 2010 decision of the Constitutional Court, by which all methods of involuntary commitment previewed under French law were declared unconstitutional (Troisoeufs & Eyraud, 2015). In the 1980s, the first association of people diagnosed with mental health conditions focusing on defending the rights of patients, *L'Association des Psychotiques Stabilisés Autonomes* (APSA), was founded with the support of psychiatrists. The first patient group with a specific focus on advocacy, *Advocacy France*, only came into being in the 1990s, drawing inspiration from advocacy groups in the US (Laval, 2015). Nevertheless, most French self-help and support groups still focus primarily on the provision of support and education for people diagnosed and their families (Troisoeufs & Eyraud, 2015). Such groups became all the more popular after the law stipulating the creation of mutual help groups—*Groupes d'Entraide Mutuelle* (GEMs)—was adopted in 2005. By 2008, 300 GEMs had developed (Girard, 2008), and in 2016, 430 GEMs were counted throughout the French territories (CNSA, 2017). Nevertheless, most of them continue to function locally, they do not reach the broad public, and have little political influence.

In the US, the peer support movement has its origins in the practices of hiring people diagnosed with mental health conditions in asylums and other psychiatric institutions in the 1920s (McCosker, 2018). The focus on self-help acquired impetus due to the popularity of psychoanalytic approaches in this country and its espousal of dominant American values, such as individual self-determination and entrepreneurialism. Under its influence, the self came to be perceived as an ongoing project, as malleable, adjustable, and improvable. And a lot of attention started to be paid to the development of behavioral approaches in mental healthcare, meant to help people diagnosed with mental health conditions better "cope" and "adjust" (Illlouz, 2008). Self-help and support groups in this country have their origin in two different types of organizations. Thus, self-help groups are linked to the funding of Alcoholics Anonymous (AA) in 1935, from which self-help groups have borrowed important organizational as well as ideological elements. In 1948, the first Fountain House, a social club for people diagnosed with mental health conditions, was founded in New York by We Are Not Alone, a group of ex-patients from the State Hospital. In the 1950s, the Fountain House came under the leadership of a social worker and broadened its focus to include, next to socialization, employment training, so that its members could gain and retain jobs (Dincin, 1975). This model has spread and thrived over the years, now counting clubhouses across the US, the UK, and Scandinavia. One of the first instances of support groups in the US is Recovery Inc., which was founded by neuropsychiatrist Abraham Low in 1937 in Chicago, to care for people with mental health conditions after their discharge from hospital. While soon thereafter Recovery Inc. also turned into a self-help group, its success has been more modest compared to AA and other similar groups.

These developments took place in a context marked by calls to reform mental health hospitals and turn them from places of confinement into spaces of care. They were also informed by the growing realization that the availability and accessibility of community care provisions were insufficient due to the rapid pace of de-institutionalization, ensuing organizational loopholes, and insufficient funding (Brown, 1988; Estroff, 1985/2001). Support groups and self-help groups thus became popular at a time when different expectations were being formulated about the relations between medical professionals and people diagnosed, and when new types of professionals and more social actors were becoming engaged in the provision of mental healthcare services (Norman, 2006). The 1980s inaugurated a lasting period of proliferation and diversification for self-help and (mutual) support groups in the US. For instance, a national survey conducted in 2002 revealed that there were 7467 organizations led by and for consumers of mental health services and their families, a substantial number compared to the 4546 traditional, professional-led mental health organizations (Goldstrom et al., 2006). In recent years, many self-help and support groups have also proliferated and diversified online (Kaufman & Whitehead, 2016) and the active role of "informed supporters" (Barak et al., 2009), that is, people diagnosed with the same mental health condition, in helping others with the same diagnosis by providing them with "more tailored feedback" (Barak et al., 2009:8) has become widely acknowledged. These activities have been shaped by the ways in which the provision of mental healthcare has been organized in the US and France, and by the challenges experienced by the mental healthcare systems in both countries, which I now briefly describe.

Mental Healthcare in the US and France

The development of different types of mental healthcare expertise and the dominant approaches to the study of mental health conditions also reverberated in the ways in which mental healthcare was provided. While asylums and psychiatric hospitals continued to be the main institutions focusing on the diagnosis and treatment of people diagnosed with mental health conditions throughout the first half of the twentieth century, important changes started to take place in the 1960s. In France, psychiatric expertise came under heavy criticism and mental healthcare came to be organized in sectors, with each sector providing care to roughly 70,000 adult inhabitants (Verdoux, 2003; Verdoux & Tignol, 2003). Developed largely in response to calls for reform made by the antipsychiatry movement (Castel, 1981), the sector was designed as a means through which mental healthcare could be provided by a multidisciplinary team of professionals headed by a psychiatrist. This team was expected to be familiar with the community and to be able to guide and assist the patient's reintegration, thereby importantly ensuring continuity of care (Coldefy, 2007; Petitjean, 2009). The events of May 1968 also marked a turning point for the standing of psychoanalysis in France, as it came to be widely adopted, both as a therapeutic approach and as a cultural phenomenon (Turkle, 1981).

In contrast, in the US, psychoanalysis was the object of criticism by the antipsychiatry movement along with psychiatry (Turkle, 1981) due to its medicalization and close integration in dominant institutions (Illlouz, 2008). In 1963 the Community Mental Health Act was signed in the US, which significantly changed the provision of mental healthcare through the establishment of community mental health centers throughout the country. As people diagnosed who had been previously treated in asylums and hospitals could receive mental healthcare services within their communities, this set into motion the process of de-institutionalization. Economic considerations played an important part in these developments, as the availability of new medications and therapeutic approaches rendered mental healthcare in the community more cost-effective. The process of deinstitutionalization unfolded at a higher rate in the last few decades of the twentieth century, which led to new challenges for people diagnosed with health conditions and mental health professionals.

Even though the process of de-institutionalization was meant to improve the provision of mental healthcare and render it economical, over the last few decades, the French and the American healthcare systems have found themselves in a precarious state. In France, most citizens are insured and have free access to mental healthcare in the public sector. Although at the beginning of the twenty-first century, the French healthcare system was voted the best out of 191 nations (WHO, 2000), such an extraordinary ranking came at a very high cost. In 2013, for instance, roughly 10.9% of the country's GDP was allocated to the health sector (OECD Health Statistics, 2015). In the field of mental healthcare more specifically, the French government has been confronted with multiple challenges, leading researchers and journalists to note at various moments in time that French psychiatry was in crisis (Castel, 1981; Coffin, 2009; Pignarre, 2006) or that it was experiencing a "severe depression" (Le Monde, 2018). In 2008, mental health conditions represented about 32% of the country's overall disease burden (WHO, 2008) and their incidence has been steadily increasing (OECD, 2016), thereby placing tremendous pressure on the mental healthcare system. For instance, in 2016, 2.1 million patients were admitted either to one of the 3900 centers of medico-psychological expertise spread throughout France or to psychiatric hospitals (about 25%).

Although the process of deinstitutionalization has occurred at a much slower rate in France than in other countries (Petitjean, 2009), over the last three decades the number of hospital beds available for people diagnosed with mental health conditions has been reduced by 70%. Most of the state's budget for mental health continues, however, to be allocated to in-hospital forms of treatment (OECD, 2016; Petitjean, 2009), while outpatient alternatives are insufficient. Furthermore, the centers of medico-psychological expertise, which were developed along with the sector as a link between general practitioners and psychiatric hospitals, have been the victims of several restructuring measures brought about by reforms that will be discussed in more detail in the following chapter. The lack of personnel and other resources has thus led to considerable delays in the provision of mental healthcare, as individuals experiencing symptoms may wait up to one year before having a first appointment, and has challenged the monitoring and timely modifications of treatment for the already registered patients. Furthermore, since the psychoanalytical model remained the dominant approach to mental health until the 2000s, some claim that the French mental healthcare system is characterized by "underdevelopment in community psychiatry, accessibility of mental health professionals trained in cognitive-behavioral psychotherapy, and psychiatric research" (Verdoux, 2003:85). Yet others criticize the "scientism" currently characterizing dominant approaches in the provision of mental healthcare in France and deplore the decline of psychoanalysis as the demise of one of the last "humanistic" approaches focusing on the individual within the full context of his/her own life (Roudinesco, 2019).

The discrepancies noted in terms of the availability of asylums at the beginning of this chapter resonate nowadays with significant differences between regions regarding the resources at their disposal, the distribution of outpatient clinics, and the number of existing mental hospitals (Coldefy et al., 2009; Coldefy, 2007; Provost & Bauer, 2001; Verdoux, 2003). The distribution of medical professionals is also skewed, with rural areas (Coldefy, 2007) and regions in Northern France (Petitjean, 2009; Verdoux, 2003) struggling due to a low number of specialists. Furthermore, while France was once the country with one of the highest number of psychiatrists in the world, their amount has been decreasing steadily, not only as the result of measures meant to render the provision of mental healthcare more efficient, but also because of the unpopularity of psychiatry as a specialization among young doctors. Thus, since 2012, the internship positions available in psychiatry have no longer been filled, with a turn for the worse signaled in 2019, when 17% of positions remained vacant, and only a minor improvement booked in 2020, when 11% of positions remained unoccupied (Raybaud, 2021). This is bound to affect people diagnosed with bipolar disorder or in need of such a diagnosis, since in France the diagnosis, treatment, and evaluation of the condition's evolution are determined by psychiatrists. General practitioners (GPs) play a different role, as they function as first points of contact and subsequently as the ones who administer the treatment and who are frequently in touch with the patients.

The American mental healthcare system has also been confronted with important challenges (Boyle & Callahan, 1995). Unlike in France, deinstitutionalization occurred in the US at a very high rate. Yet, few solutions were put in place to enable people diagnosed to receive the care they needed within the community (Estroff, 1985/2001), and not many people knew about them, when such solutions existed (Grob, 2005). The situation worsened toward the turn of the century, prompting the chair of the President's New Freedom Commission on Mental Health to state in 2002 that "the system needs dramatic reform because it is incapable of efficiently delivering and financing effective treatments—such as medications, psychotherapies, and other services—that have taken decades to develop. Responsibility for these services is scattered among agencies, programs, and levels of government" (Hogan, in Gijswijt-Hofstra, 2002:156f). The delivery of cost-effective mental healthcare services continues to remain a problem, as spending has been increasing at alarming rates. In 2019, $225 billion was dedicated to this sector, marking an increase of 52% compared to the expenditure in 2009 (Open Minds Market Intelligence Report, 2019). At the same time, the delivery of mental healthcare continues to remain highly fragmented and insurance companies often distinguish between medical and behavioral types of interventions, prompting differences in facilities, data collection systems, and reimbursement requirements (Mou & Insel, 2021).

While some American people diagnosed with mental health conditions nowadays receive better quality care than they would have a few decades earlier, the system continues to be marked by important inequalities. Even though the passage of the Affordable Care Act has enabled more individuals to have access to healthcare, over 10% of the people diagnosed with mental health conditions continue to be uninsured (Mental Health America, 2022). Furthermore, the quality of care varies depending on one's type of insurance. For instance, the coverage provided by Medicare is limited, as it only enables access to about 25% of the mental healthcare professionals registered in the US. Moreover, it allows for a total of 190 days of in-hospital psychiatric care, even for people diagnosed with severe mental health conditions, such as bipolar disorder. At the same time, only 56% of psychiatrists accept commercial insurances (Leonhardt, 2021). As a consequence, not all insured people diagnosed with mental health conditions have access to the same type of treatment (Hogan, 2003), with evidence indicating that the mental healthcare received by members of ethnic minorities continues to be limited and of lower quality (National Institute on Minority Health and Disparities, 2019; Kataoka et al., 2002).

There are also significant geographic differences in terms of access to mental healthcare, which echoes somewhat the situation in France. Thus, in different states, mental healthcare services are reimbursed to varying degrees, and managed care controls limit access to costly services while seeking to promote cheaper options more widely (Scheid, 2000). Not only does the availability of community services differ, but the system is also marked by important discrepancies regarding the number and type of medical professionals available (Mental Health Care Professional Shortage Areas (HPSAs), 2020), with more than 112 million Americans living nowadays in areas with few mental healthcare providers (Leonhardt, 2021). Thus, while in New York, Massachusetts, and Vermont there are more than 15 psychiatrists per 100,000 people, in Texas and Idaho there are fewer than 6 (Simon, 2015). Furthermore, there appear to be over 4000 areas across the US with only one psychiatrist for 30,000 people (Simon, 2015). These issues are further complicated by the fact that the overall number of psychiatrists available is bound to decrease over the coming years. This is due to a diminished interest among young medical doctors to specialize in psychiatry and to the upcoming retirement of a large number of psychiatrists, as 59% of them are 55 or older (National Council for Mental Wellbeing, 2017; Simon, 2015). In this context, matters are not made any easier by differences in legislation among states, which prevent mental healthcare practitioners from practicing everywhere in the US.

It is against this background that the Internet and, more recently, the development and spread of digital and AI-based technologies have led to great hopes that they may enhance the accessibility and quality of mental healthcare, both in the US and in France. At the same time, these technologies have also given rise to grave concerns about their potential to further inequalities and fragmentation. It is to these utopian and dystopian expectations that I now turn.

Digital and AI-Based Technologies in Mental Healthcare

A plethora of digital technologies, such as smart phones, smart clothes, smart pills, and wearables, contribute these days to the collection of different types of data and inform new hopes about the provision of mental healthcare (Bhugra et al., 2017; Bradstreet et al., 2019; Flore, 2021; Gooding, 2019; Mou & Insel, 2021; Pickersgill, 2019). For instance, a broad variety of stakeholders, ranging from governmental representatives[1] to medical professionals and members of the industry, believe that "automation using digital technology could improve the delivery and quality of care in psychiatry, and reduce costs" (Bauer et al., 2019:338). While many AI-based technologies are still at the stage of prototypes, the implementation and widespread use of digital technologies is bound to contribute to important changes in the understanding and approach to expertise about mental health. A review of recent publications that I have undertaken indicates that these technologies are expected to play a role in three main areas: (1) the identification of biomarkers, so that mental health conditions can be diagnosed earlier and more reliably; (2) the personalization of therapeutic approaches based on individual characteristics and the comprehensive and continuous monitoring of people diagnosed; and (3) the provision of existing treatment in new ways and the development of novel therapeutic approaches.

The search for objective criteria to establish mental health diagnoses, which started in the early days of the asylum, continues nowadays through the use of AI-based technologies. Thus, machine-learning algorithms are currently being trained in collaboration with psychiatrists to identify people with various mental health diagnoses at a prodromal stage, when symptoms have not yet manifested themselves clearly (Bauer et al., 2019; Miller, 2019; Rudin & Ustun, 2018; Shatte et al., 2019). Promising in this sense are various natural language processing algorithms, which are meant to analyze linguistic as well as paralinguistic aspects to help in diagnosis as well as in the prediction of an upcoming mental health

---

[1] In the US, the Department of Veterans Affairs and Department of Defense has developed mental health apps (lagan et al., 2020).

episode. It is thus hoped that patterns of speech, one's vocabulary, as well as acoustic elements can be rendered legible as mental health markers and indicators. As we have seen in the first section of this chapter, a lot of attention has traditionally been paid to these elements in psychiatric expertise. What is new here, however, is the breadth and level of precision and granularity with which these elements are monitored, recorded, and assessed. This is often invoked as a cause for celebration by the technological companies involved in such developments, as the following quote illustrates: "With AI, our words will be a window into our mental health" (IBM, 2017).

Next to the development of reliable and objective criteria for diagnosis, the correct and timely identification of mood states has also received a lot of attention. Growing efforts have been made to combine digital behavior indicators with physiological data, and to link various patterns of engagement with digital technologies, such as the intensity and speed of smartphone keystrokes, the number and content of social media posts, and variations in voice patterns, with specific mood episodes. Thus, next to linguistic markers and voice analysis, elements of one's interactions with digital technologies are transformed into potential mental health symptoms. Such digital phenotyping[2] (Martinez-Martin et al., 2018) is also expected to contribute to a better understanding of an individual's reaction to a particular treatment and to increased treatment adherence.

The use of digital technologies in the provision of existing therapeutic approaches has been accompanied by visions whereby significant changes are operated in the frequency, length, and content of such therapies. For instance, proponents of Ecological Momentary Interventions (EMIs) have advocated for the provision of multiple psychological interventions or behavioral prompts spread throughout the day and informed by sensory data acquired through digital technologies (D'Alfonso, 2020). This way, the delivery of personalized therapy is understood as not only being attuned to a specific person, but also as adjustable to the particular context in which that person may find him/herself in and to the best timing

---

[2] Digital phenotyping is used by clinicians with the aim of creating objective parameters that correlate with diagnostic criteria by using extensive data about a person to refine diagnosis and predict behavior. It is a form of population monitoring/surveillance.

when it should be provided or ingested. There are also technologies which aim for the personalization of therapeutic interventions by facilitating common decision-making. Such technologies elicit information about each person's preferences, needs, and values and subsequently make it available to medical professionals, so that they can decide about the best medical treatment based, ideally, on a richer understanding of the person's symptoms, challenges, life circumstances, and goals. An example of such a digital decision-making aid is common ground, which was shaped by the experiential knowledge of its developer, who is allegedly diagnosed with a mental health condition. Importantly, many also hope that AI-based technologies will enable the development of novel therapeutic interventions based on an individual's genes, lifestyle, and other relevant environmental markers (Fernandes et al., 2017), thereby turning precision psychiatric medicine into a reality.

Digital and AI-based technologies have also contributed to changes in how already available therapeutic approaches are provided and by whom. Thus, the use of computers for the provision of various mental health services ranging from online chats to text messaging between people diagnosed with mental health conditions and medical professionals or other people diagnosed is widespread. Videoconferencing tools are being increasingly used to arrange mental healthcare appointments both in the US and in France, as many technological companies have started to develop technologies to address the geographic disparities in the provision of mental healthcare discussed above and to help save time for both mental healthcare practitioners and the people diagnosed. For instance, Doctolib, which is the current leader of digital healthcare services in France, as it comprises 80% of this market, launched a smartphone application in January 2019. The application allows people diagnosed with mental health conditions or experiencing symptoms to book video consultations with mental healthcare professionals of their choice, regardless of where they find themselves (Blaquière, 2019). The intention is to enhance convenience for both parties, as the times and dates at which different mental healthcare professionals are available are clearly indicated. While only medical professionals have to pay for the use of Doctolib and its application, in the US people diagnosed are required to pay for online counseling services, but many of them, such as BetterHelp and Talkspace, are currently reimbursed by some insurance companies.

Chatbots are also becoming increasingly popular not only for mood tracking, but also for the provision of cognitive-behavioral therapy, mindfulness, and behavioral reinforcement. Of notoriety in France is the application My Sherpa, developed by Doctorpsy, which is claimed to have been downloaded by over 220,000 people. It allows people experiencing various mental health issues to access psychotherapy and to interact with a chatbot about their mental states. In the US and many other countries, numerous services are provided by three of the most prominent chatbots in mental healthcare—Tess, Wysa, and Woebot. Chatbots are seen as viable solutions for people diagnosed with mental health conditions who may have difficulties accessing conventional therapeutic services, and who may appreciate the constant availability of such "therapist robots" and their supposedly neutral, non-judgmental character. Furthermore, "machine counselors" have also been used rather successfully in suicide prevention services, and great hopes are attached to virtual therapeutic agents using avatar representations, such as ELLIE, which are meant to move beyond language processing and to engage in the analysis of nonverbal signals.

Digital and AI-based technologies are not only expected to contribute to better diagnosis and treatment, but also expected to bring about important changes in the work of medical professionals and in their relations to people diagnosed. For instance, many hope AI will help improve the quality of care by reducing clinicians' paperwork-related workload and by summarizing important information from a person's patient record. Whereas monitoring devices are often discussed in relation to acquiring insights into people's physical and mood states, some have also been implemented to keep an eye on the mental healthcare provided by professionals. For instance, in the US "Electronic Visit Verification" is used to log in the precise duration of home visits by mental health service providers (Olowu, 2015). Importantly, the widespread use of digital technologies in mental health may be accompanied by the blurring of numerous categories, given their more malleable character. For instance, depending on the context of use, a digital pill may be a digital treatment, but it may also be a form of surveillance or control (Cosgrove et al.,

2020). Such blurring of boundaries may lead to challenges for the ways in which expertise is performed, and may require new sets of skills to navigate the changes they may bring to the relations between people diagnosed and mental healthcare professionals. It may also require both groups to acquire greater insights into the available legislation, in order to better understand how such technologies and the data acquired through them can be used and shared.

Whereas proponents of AI and digital technologies in mental healthcare are enthusiastic about the transformations their implementation could lead to, critics have drawn attention to some problematic aspects regarding their (future) use (Fiske et al., 2019). Since many of these concerns are also valid in relation to the data currently collected from online platforms such as those that this book focuses on, they will be discussed in more detail, as they are important to consider when engaging with the insights provided in the next chapters. The main types of criticism identified focus on the feasibility and efficiency of the collaborations required, the quality of the data, and the epistemic character of the insights that can be derived through the use of digital technologies. Thus, some commentators (Carr, 2020; Pasquale, 2020) have emphasized that the responsible and reliable development, assessment, and implementation of such technologies require the collaboration of a diverse community of experts, including researchers, clinicians, regulators, and people diagnosed. This is bound to be an arduous process, as the development of a common understanding, familiarity with core approaches in each discipline, new research methods, and novel ways to redistribute responsibility will likely be required.

Other scholars have raised concerns about the type of data that can be obtained and from whom and the consequences this may lead to. Thus, the data that are currently collected through monitoring devices and used to train algorithms that are supposed to help in decision-making do not (sufficiently) capture personal, social, cultural, and economic factors, yet these importantly shape one's mental state (Birk & Samuel, 2020; Bradstreet et al., 2019). This situation is partly due to the quantitative logic underlying these technologies, as they mainly record aspects that can be measured and analyzed through statistical methods. At the same time, it is also informed by the biological language surrounding digital pheno-typing, which orients attention in particular directions and may thus lead to the reification of mental health conditions as biological (Birk & Samuel, 2020). From this point of view, Bemme et al. (2020, not paginated) convincingly warned that "[t]he quest for holism through big data may thus lead to a re-emergence of the tyranny of reductionism." Apart from the decontextualization and reductionism that might be operated through digital data collection practices, scholars have also warned about important inequalities among people diagnosed with mental health conditions in terms of access and representation. While in the days of the asylum, mostly the poor and the destitute were overrepresented in the data collected (Porter, 2018), nowadays socioeconomic status and location inform the availability of data, as almost half of the world's population still does not have access to the Internet and digital technologies. Another problematic aspect is that thus far people diagnosed with mental health conditions and their carers have not been involved in the development of AI-based interventions (Bradstreet et al., 2019). Bradstreet et al. (2019:128) warned in this sense that "[t]here are risks of replicating existing and even creating new inequalities in health and mental health as well as risks that new forms of coercion or compulsory treatment could emerge. Scrutiny, transparency and algorithmic accountability are essential."

Noteworthy concerns have also been raised about the epistemic character of the insights acquired from such data and the validity of the decisions based on them. For instance, critics have highlighted that algorithms are trained on insights acquired through the subjective and selective work of human professionals. From this point of view, algorithms are not objective, as they reflect current hierarchies of knowledge and patterns of exploitation in their functioning (Bemme et al., 2020). Another relevant perspective is provided by Coghlan and D'Alfonso (2021), who put forward four types of possible relations between the information generated using digital devices and mental health phenomena: two types of causal relations, a correlative and a constitutive relation. Through these four scenarios, Coghlan and D'Alfonso (2021) show that the availability of data collected through digital technologies does not automatically lead to reliable insights about people's mental health. To arrive at the latter, inferences need to be made and their quality depends on the availability of accurate and precise definitions, adequate measurement tools, the possibility to correctly identify distorting effects, and the opportunity to draw upon additional types of data. Thus, while digital phenotyping may contribute to new and more reliable knowledge about mental health, caution is needed not to misinterpret and misrepresent the epistemic character of the data collected through digital technologies. This is particularly important, given that algorithms have thus far had a hard time distinguishing between different disease categories from the same data, while people diagnosed with mental health conditions present a high level of comorbidity (Birk & Samuel, 2020).

Criticism regarding the use of AI and digital technologies in mental healthcare has also focused on the changes they have prompted to the ways in which the psychiatric subject can be constituted and studied. In this sense, scholars have highlighted the blurring of boundaries between those who make and who are made by the data collected through such tools. They have also argued that the real-time collection of different types of psychological data and the countless possibilities to aggregate them contribute to the development of an "aggregate human" that defies stable categories as well as micro and macro distinctions (Bemme et al., 2020). This raises questions about the types of mental healthcare that would be appropriate for such a human and about the methods through which s/he can best be studied.

Other scholars have noted the relatively narrow domain of application of these digital technologies, as most technological companies have focused their investments on tools meant to alleviate mild to moderate symptoms and have manifested less interest for the development of instruments able to address the more severe symptoms of conditions such as bipolar disorder or schizophrenia. This way, those who most need mental healthcare services might be further disadvantaged and the widespread use of digital tools will most likely fail to contribute to curbing current mental healthcare costs (Mou & Insel, 2021). Furthermore, considerable doubts have also been expressed about the quality of the therapeutic approaches enabled through these technologies, as several reviews have indicated that many of the technologies and applications that people diagnosed with mental health conditions can access freely or at a low cost have not been scientifically tested or have only been assessed through short, small-scale studies.

Whereas numerous mobile phone applications are available for use for people diagnosed with various mental health conditions (Faurholt-Jepsen et al., 2018; Faurholt-Jepsen et al., 2019) and are downloaded millions of times per month (Marathe & Ravi, 2020; Nicholas et al., 2015), their quality can vary widely and they are much less regulated than medicine-based treatments. Furthermore, since most information available thus far consists of engagement metrics, there is limited understanding about the ways in which these technologies shape the quality of mental healthcare care. While some people diagnosed may feel empowered to use digital technologies to better understand and manage their conditions, others may feel overwhelmed. Important questions have also been raised about the long-term impact of such technologies on people's abilities to manage their mental health, with some critics worrying that intensive engagement with digital technologies may lead to "de-skilling," as individuals would come to rely more on these tools and spend less time and effort actively managing their condition. Thus, even in the case of applications and digital technologies of proven quality, it is unclear how to optimally deploy them in practice, and how the preferences of individuals diagnosed with mental health conditions and the specificity of their daily lives could best be considered in this sense.

Numerous critics have also raised concerns about various legal and regulatory aspects in regard to the use of digital technologies. Thus, many commentators have highlighted the highly intrusive character of these devices (Carr, 2020), as they imply continuous video and audio monitoring, which makes their acceptability questionable. In this sense, Guta et al. (2018) argued that such technologies should be seen as part of a "larger integrated surveillance apparatus" or of a "digital medicine panopticon," which focuses on already marginalized communities. People diagnosed with mental health conditions enjoy different degrees of legal protection in this sense, depending on the country they live in. For instance, in France and other countries of the European Union, the General Data Protection Regulation (GDPR) should afford them greater protection, whereas in the US the legal provisions available remain limited and differ among states. Other critics (Carr, 2020) have raised concerns about the degree to which people diagnosed with mental health conditions, whose state can fluctuate over time, can give informed consent and about the time frame within which such consent could be considered valid. Another important concern stems from the fact that data collected through such technologies could become available to third parties who may use it in a discriminatory fashion or in other ways disadvantageous to the individuals from which they have been collected. Such data are already collected and used in the judiciary, as some people with mental health conditions who would otherwise be hospitalized or incarcerated are allowed to stay home under GPS monitoring (Boone et al., 2017). While at first glance such digital approaches may seem more humane and affording better care, there are also concerns that they may entail new types of coercive measures, including the mandatory sharing of mental healthcare information, such as the number of hospitalizations or suicidal behavior, across institutions. Some commentators therefore expect digital technologies to be intensively used in coercive psychiatric interventions (Gooding, 2019).

The developments described here sketch the conditions of possibility for the epistemic practices that this book focuses on. The online performances of expertise about bipolar disorder to which we will now turn our attention carry therefore vestiges of the different theoretical approaches that shaped the development of knowledge about mental health, of the various tools and instruments used for the collection of data that have been discussed in the first part of this chapter. They are also shaped by the new practices and forms of knowledge that digital technologies currently allow for and by the hopes and fears that AI-based technologies have generated among different stakeholders. How expertise about bipolar disorder is performed in this context by official bodies in the US and France is discussed at length in the following chapter.

References

American Psychiatric Association. (2013). Diagnostic and Statistical Manual of Mental Disorders, fifth edition (DSM-5).

American Psychiatric Association. (1968). Diagnostic and Statistical Manual of Mental Disorders, second edition (DSM-II).

Arribas-Ayllon, M., Bartlett, A., & Lewis, J. (2019). Psychiatric Genetics. From Hereditary Madness to Big Biology. Routledge.

Barak, A., Klein, B., & Proudfoot, J. (2009). Defining Internet-Supported Therapeutic Interventions. *Annals of Behavioral Medicine, 38*(1), 4–17.

Baron, M., Risch, N., Hamburger, R., et al. (1987). Genetic Linkage between X- chromosome Markers And Bipolar Affective Illness. *Nature, 326*, 289–292.

Bauer, M., Monteith, S., Geddes, J., Gitlin, M. J., Grof, P., Whybrow, P. C., & Glenn, T. (2019). Automation to Optimise Physician Treatment of Individual Patients: Examples in Psychiatry. *The Lancet Psychiatry, 6*(4), 338–349.

Bemme, D., Brenman, N., & Semel, B. (2020, October 13). The Subjects of Digital Psychiatry'. *Somatosphere*. Available at http://somatosphere.net/2020/subjects-of-digital-psychiatry.html/.

Bernadet, P., Douraki, T., & Vaillant, C. (2002). *Psychiatrie, Droits de l'Homme et Défense des Usagers en Europe*. Écrès.

Bhugra, D., Tasman, A., Pathare, S., Priebe, S., Smith, S., Torous, J., et al. (2017). The WPA-Lancet Psychiatry Commission on the Future of Psychiatry. *The Lancet Psychiatry, 4*(10), 775–818.

Birk, R., & Samuel, G. (2020). Can Digital Data Diagnose Mental Health Problems? A Sociological Exploration of 'Digital Phenotyping'. *Sociology of Health & Illness, 42*(8), 1873–1887.

Blaquière, J. (2019, January 14). Doctolib se lance dans la téléconsultation. *Le Figaro*. Available at https://www.lefigaro.fr/societes/2019/01/14/20005-20190114ARTFIG 00128-doctolib-se-lance-dans-la-teleconsultation.php

Boone, M., van der Kooij, M., & Rap, S. (2017). The Highly Reintegrative Approach of Electronic Monitoring in the Netherlands. *European Journal of Probation, 9*(1), 46–61.

Boyle, P., & Callahan, D. (1995). Managed Care in Mental Health: The Ethical Issues. *Health Affairs, 14*, 7–23.

Bradstreet, S., Allan, S., & Gumley, A. (2019). Adverse Event Monitoring in mHealth for Psychosis Interventions Provides an Important Opportunity for Learning. *Journal of Mental Health, 28*(5), 461–466.

Brown, P. (1988). *The Transfer of Care: Psychiatric Deinstitutionalization and Its Aftermath*. Routledge Kegan & Paul.

Caisse Nationale de Solidarité pour l'Autonomie (CNSA) (2017, Mai). Les GEM. Groupes d'entraide mutuelle. *Les cahiers pédagogiques de la CNSA*.

Carr, S. (2020). 'AI gone mental': Engagement and Ethics in Data-driven Technology for Mental Health. *Journal of Mental Health, 29*(2), 125–130.

Castel, R. (1981). *La Gestion des Risques. De l'Anti-Psychiatrie à l'Après-Psychanalyse*. Minuit.

Coffin, J.-C. (2009). La Psychiatrie par Temps de Crise. *Études, 6*(410), 751–761.

Coghlan, S., & D'Alfonso, S. (2021). Digital Phenotyping: An Epistemic and Methodological Analysis. *Philosophy & Technology, 34*(4), 1905–1928.

Coldefy, M. (Ed.). (2007). *La Prise en Charge de la Santé Mentale. Recueil d'Études Statistiques*. La Documentation Française.

Coldefy, M., Le Fur, P., Lucas-Gabrielli, V., & Mousquès, J. (2009). Une Mise en Perspective de l'Offre de Soins des Secteurs de Psychiatrie Générale et du Recours à la Medicine Générale. *Pratiques et Organization des Soins, 40*(3), 197–206.

Cosgrove, L., Karter, J., McGinley, M., & Morrill, Z. (2020). Digital Phenotyping and Digital Psychotropic Drugs: Mental Health Surveillance Tools That Threaten Human Rights. *Health and Human Rights, 22*(2), 33–39.

D'Alfonso, S. (2020). AI and Mental Health. *Current Opinion in Psychology, 36*, 112–117.

Dincin, J. (1975). Psychiatric Rehabilitation. *Schizophrenia Bulletin, 13*, 131–147.

Egeland, J. A., Gerhard, D. S., Pauls, D. L., et al. (1987). Bipolar Affective Disorder Linked to DNA Markers on Chromosome 11. *Nature, 325*, 783–787.

Estroff S (1985/2001) Making it Crazy. An Ethnography of Psychiatric Clients in an American Community 2nd ed. : University of California Press.

Faurholt-Jepsen, M., Bauer, M., & Kessing, L. (2018). Smartphone-Based Objective Monitoring in Bipolar Disorder: Status and Considerations. *International Journal of Bipolar Disorders, 6*, 6.

Faurholt-Jepsen, M., Torri, E., Cobo, J., et al. (2019). Smart-phone based Self-monitoring in Bipolar Disorder: Evaluation of Usability and Feasibility of Two Systems. *Journal of Bipolar Disorders, 7*(1), 1–11.

Fernandes, B. S., Williams, L. M., Steiner, J., Leboyer, M., Carvalho, A. F., & Berk, M. (2017). The New Field of 'Precision Psychiatry. *BMC Medicine, 15*(1), 80.

Fiske, A., Henningsen, P., & Buyx, A. (2019). Your Robot Therapist Will See You Now: Ethical Implications of Embodied Artificial Intelligence in Psychiatry, Psychology, and Psychotherapy. *Journal of Medical Internet Research, 21*(5), 1–12.

Flore, J. (2021). Ingestible Sensors, Data, and Pharmaceuticals: Subjectivity in the Era of Digital Mental Health. *New Media & Society*, 1–18.

Foucault M (1972/2010). *History of Madness*. : Routledge. Translated by Jonathan Murphy and Jean Khalfa.

Freud S (1917/2005) On Murder, Mourning and Melancholia. : Penguin Books. Trans. by Shaun Whiteside

Girard, V. (2008). Dossier n° 13- Auto Support en Santé Mentale en France. *Bulletin Amades, 75*, 1–9.

Goldstrom, I., Campbell, J., Rogers, J., Lambert, D., Blacklow, B., Hendeseon, M., & Manderscheid, R. (2006). National Estimates for Mental Health Mutual Support Groups, Self-Help Organizations, and Consumer-Operated Services. *Administration and Policy in Mental Health and Mental Health Services Research, 33*(1), 92–103.

Gooding, P. (2019). Mapping the Rise of Digital Mental Health Technologies: Emerging Issues for Law and Society. *International Journal of Law and Psychiatry, 67*, 1–11.

Grob, G. (2005). The Transformation of Mental Health Policy in Twentieth-Century America. In M. Gijswijt-Hofstra, H. Oosterhuis, J. Vijselaar, & H. Freeman (Eds.), *Psychiatry and Mental Health Care in the Twentieth-Century: Comparisons and Approaches* (pp. 141–161). Amsterdam University Press.

Guta, A., Voronka, J., & Gagnon, M. (2018). Resisting the Digital Medicine Panopticon: Toward a Bioethics of the Oppressed. *The American Journal of Bioethics, 18*(9), 62–64.

Healy, D. (2008). *Mania: A Short History of Bipolar Disorder*. John Hopkins University Press.

Hochmann, J. (2017). *Histoire de la Psychiatrie. Paris: Presses Universitaires de France* (4th ed.).

Hogan, M. (2003). The President's New Freedom Commission: Recommen dations to Transform Mental Health Care in America. *Psychiatric Services, 54*(11), 1467–1474.

Hogan, M., & to President George W Bush. (2002). Interim Report of the President's New Freedom Commission on Mental Health. In M. Gijswijt-Hofstra, H. Oosterhuis, J. Vijselaar, & H. Freeman (Eds.), *Psychiatric Cultures Compared. Psychiatry and Mental Health Care* (p. 156). Amsterdam University Press.

IBM Research Editorial Staff (January 5, 2017). 'IBM 5 in 5: With AI, our words will be a window into our mental health.' Retrieved from: https://www.ibm.com/blogs/research/2017/01/ibm-5-in-5-our-words-will-be-the-windows-to-our-mental-health/. Accessed on 23.09.2021

Illlouz, E. (2008). *Saving the Modern Soul. Therapy, Emotions, and the Culture of Self-Help*. University of California Press.

Kataoka, S., Zhang, L., & Wells, K. (2002). Unmet Need for Mental Health Care Among U.S. Children: Variation by Ethnicity and Insurance Status. *American Journal of Psychiatry, 159*, 1548–1555.

Kaufman, S., & Whitehead, K. (2016). Producing, Ratifying, and Resisting Support in an Online Support Forum. *Health*, 1–17. Advance online publication. https://doi.org/10.1177/1363459315628043

Lagan, S., Ramakrishnan, A., Lamont, E. *et al.* (2020). Digital Health Developments and Drawbacks: A Review and Analysis of Top-Returned Apps for Bipolar Disorder. *Int J Bipolar Disord, 8*, 39. https://doi.org/10.1186/s40345-020-00202-4

Laval, C. (2015). Edito. *Rhizome, 58*(4), 1–2.

Le Monde. (2018, August 18). *La Psychiatrie, un secteur en état d'urgence.* Available at https://www.lemonde.fr/idees/article/2018/08/18/la-psychiatrie-un-secteur-en-etat-d-urgence_5343765_3232.html

Leonhardt, M. (2021, May 10). *What You Need to Know About the Cost and Accessibility of Mental Health Care in America.* Available at https://www.cnbc.com/2021/05/10/cost-and-accessibility-of-mental-health-care-in-america.html

Marathe, P., & Ravi, S. (2020, December 8). The Mental Health Dilemma: If Technology is the Problem, Can it also be the Solution?. *STAT News.* Available at https://www.statnews.com/2020/12/08/mental-health-dilemma-technology-cause-and-solution/

Martinez-Martin, N., Insel, T., Dagum, P., Greely, H., & Cho, M. (2018). Data Mining for Health: Staking Out the Ethical Territory of Digital Phenotyping. *Npj Digital Medicine, 1*(1), Article 68.

McCosker, A. (2018). Engaging Mental Health Online: Insights from *beyondblue*'s forum influencers. *New Media & Society, 20*(12), 4748–4764.

Mental Health America. (2022). *The State of Mental Health in America.* Available at https://mhanational.org/issues/state-mental-health-america

Mental Health Care Health Professional Shortage Areas (HPSAs). (2020). Available at Mental Health Care Health Professional Shortage Areas (HPSAs) | KFF

Miller, K. (2019). A Matter of Perspective: Discrimination, bias and in- equality in AI. In T. Walsh (Ed.), *Closer to the Machine. Technical, Social, and Legal Aspects of AI.* Office of the Victorian Information Commissioner. Available at https://ovic.vic.gov.au/wp-content/uploads/2019/08/closer-to-the-machine-web.pdf

Mou, D., & Insel, R. (2021, January 19). *Startups Should Focus on Innovations that Truly Improve Mental Health.* Available at https://www.statnews.com/2021/01/19/startups-innovations-truly-improve-mental-health/

National Council for Mental Wellbeing. (2017). *The Psychiatric Shortage. Causes and Solutions.* Available at https://www.thenationalcouncil.org/wp-content/uploads/2017/03/Psychiatric-Shortage_National-Council-.pdf?daf=375ateTbd56

Nicholas, J., Larsen, M., Proudfoot, J., & Christensen, H. (2015). Mobile Apps for Bipolar Disorder: A Systematic Review of Features and Content Quality. *Journal of Medical Internet Research, 17*(8), e198.

Norman, C. (2006). The Fountain House Movement, an Alternative Rehabilitation Model for People with Mental Health Problems, Members' Descriptions of What Works. *Scandinavian Journal of Caring Science, 20*, 184–192.

OECD. (2015). *Country Note: How does health spending in FRANCE compare?* OECD Health Statistics.

OECD. (2016). *Health Policy in France. OECD Health Policy Overview.* OECD.

Olowu, A. (2015). Delivering Proof of Care at the Point of Care. How Electronic Visit Verification Can Benefit Clinicians, Home Health Workers and Patients. *Health Management Technology, 36*(4), 16.

Open Minds. (2019). *The U.S. Mental Health Market: $225.1 Billion In Spending.* Market Intelligence Report.

Pasquale, F. (2020). *New Laws of Robotics. Defending Human Expertise in the Age of AI.* The Belknap Press of Harvard University Press.

Petitjean, F. (2009). The Sectorization System in France. *International Journal of Mental Health, 38*(4), 25–38.

Pickersgill, M. (2019). Digitising Psychiatry? Sociotechnical Expectations, Performative Nominalism and Biomedical Virtue in (Digital) Psychiatric Praxis. *Sociology of Health & Illness, 41*(1), 16–30.

Pignarre, P. (2006). *Les Malheurs des Psys. Psychotropes et Médicalisation du Social.* La Découverte.

Porter, T. (2018). *Genetics in the Madhouse. The Unknown History of Human Heredity.* Princeton University Press.

Provost, D., & Bauer, A. (2001). Trends and Developments in Public Psychiatry in France since 1975. *Acta Psychiatrica Scandinavica, 104*(410), 63–68.

Raybaud, A. (2021, June 16). Chez les étudiants en medicine, la psychiatrie plus délaissée que jamais. *Le Monde.* Available at https://www.lemonde.fr/campus/article/2021/06/16/chez-les-etudiants-en-medecine-la-psychiatrie-plus-delaissee-que-jamais_6084290_4401467.html

Rose, N. (2018). *Our Psychiatric Futures.* Polity Press.

Roudinesco, E. (2019, February 8). Les psychanalystes ont contribué à leur propre déclin. *Le Monde.*

Rudin, C., & Ustun, B. (2018). Optimized Scoring Systems: Toward Trust in Machine Learning for Healthcare and Criminal Justice. *Interfaces, 48*(5), 449–466.

Scheid, T. (2000). Rethinking Professional Prerogative: Managed Mental Health Care Providers. *Sociology of Health & Illness, 22*(5), 700–719.

Shatte, A., Hutchinson, D., & Teague, S. (2019). Machine Learning in Mental Health: A Scoping Review of Methods and Applications. *Psychological Medicine, 49*, 1426–1448.

Simon, C. (2015, September 9). US Faces Severe Shortage of Psychiatrists as Demand Grows-Report. *RT News*. Accessed August 12, 2017, from https://www.rt.com/usa/314777-us-shortage-psychiatrists-demand-grows/

Swain, G. (1988). *Le Sujet de la Folie. Naissance de la Psychiatrie*. Privat.

Troisoeufs, A., & Eyraud, B. (2015). Psychiatrisés en Lutte, Usagers, Gemeurs…: Une Cartographie des Différentes Formes de Participation. *Rhizome, 58*(4), 3–4.

Turkle, S. (1981). *Psychoanalytic Politics. Freud's French Revolution*. The MIT Press.

Verdoux, H. (2003). Psychiatry in France. *International Journal of Social Psychiatry, 49*(2), 83–86.

Verdoux, H., & Tignol, J. (2003). Focus on Psychiatry in France. *British Journal of Psychiatry, 183*, 466–471.

WHO. (2000). *Health Systems: Improving Performance*. World Health Report 2000. World Health Organization.

WHO. (2008). *The Global Burden of Disease: 2004 update*. World Health Organization.

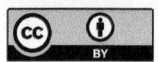

3

The Drama of Expertise About Bipolar Disorder Online

The Internet has been increasingly used by governments around the world as a cost-effective way to provide health-related information to various audiences (Barak, 1999; Bennett & Glasgow, 2009; Christensen et al., 2004; Griffiths et al., 2006; Levy & Strombeck, 2002). Whereas the US was an early enthusiast and France a relative latecomer, for almost two decades now, important governmental agencies and mental health-care providers in both countries have been sharing insights about bipolar disorder online. In so doing, they have been confronted with two major challenges. On the one hand, they need to conform with legislation requiring governmental agencies that have online platforms to make sure that the information they share online is accessible to people with disabilities. On the other hand, they are required to make their views public in a context where many people, including mental health professionals, are critical of psychiatry (Morrison, 2013), and where important struggles take place between the different types of professionals involved. This means that the official character of an institution is no longer a sufficient guarantee that the psychiatric insights it provides are accepted as knowledge, so when sharing information online, official bodies need to make proof of their expertise. Because of these challenges, "science

© The Author(s) 2023
C. Egher, *Digital Healthcare and Expertise*, Health, Technology and Society,
https://doi.org/10.1007/978-981-16-9178-2_3

communication represents a crucial activity" (Horst et al., 2017:881) nowadays and the "investigation of the Internet's applicability as a tool for public mental health interventions is important" (Ybarra & Eaton, 2005:75).

This chapter therefore focuses on the performative techniques that highly authoritative governmental agencies—*The National Institute of Mental Health* (NIMH) in the US and *La Haute Autorité de Santé* (HAS) in France—deploy to convincingly perform expertise about bipolar disorder on their online platforms. Coordination plays an important role in the development of expertise, based on the new conceptualization I put forward. Coordination can refer to how different stakeholders come to work together toward a common goal, as we shall see in the next chapter, but it also denotes the fine-tuning activities one and the same stakeholder needs to engage in across different settings, for the knowledge displayed to be authoritative. While such activities are always necessary, online they become all the more important given the multiple presences that one may have, the haphazard way in which the audience might arrive at information, and the manifold ways in which disparate elements can be linked together, thereby acquiring new meaning. This chapter focuses on this dimension of coordination and discusses the activities NIMH and HAS undertook as they had to create and manage relations across different online stages and materials (Drucker, 2011) to convincingly perform expertise about bipolar disorder online. To set the stage, I briefly discuss the context in which the American and the French governments have started to promote the use of the Internet as a cost-effective way to provide mental health-related information.

The Internet in Mental Healthcare in France and the US

As already indicated in the previous chapters, the French mental healthcare system has been undergoing substantial reforms, in order to become more cost-effective. It is against this background that the French authorities started to encourage governmental agencies and health providers to share information online both as a means to educate the general population and to facilitate collaboration between the different types of professionals involved in the provision of mental healthcare. Especially after 2012, the authorities sought to put forward online solutions to reach populations in remote areas, and to prompt people to seek help by providing them with less stigmatizing ways to become informed and to get in touch with medical professionals (eMEN, 2017). Various initiatives and pieces of legislation have facilitated these developments. Important in this sense has been the adoption in 2016 of the law for a "république numérique," which contains important regulations regarding the online provision of information, greater accessibility, personal privacy, and so on. Furthermore, building upon initiatives such as the "digital hospital program" and "Digital Patient Territories," on July 4, 2016, the French Minister of Social Affairs and Health presented the first national e-health strategy 2020 (Ministère des Affaires Sociales et de la Santé, 2016; VPH Institute, 2016), where the information, participation, and consultation of users were among the highlights. In the same year, France joined the eMEN, a six-country[1] e-mental health project meant to promote the use of innovative digital technologies in the provision of mental healthcare (eMEN, 2017).

Similarly to France, also in the US the authorities started to look for online solutions in the provision of mental healthcare out of financial considerations and because of a dramatic expected decrease in the number of psychiatrists in the near future, due to retirement and low numbers of student applications in relevant fields. It is in this context that the Internet came to be seen as an effective and relatively cheap medium that could be efficiently used (1) to educate people about mental health in an attempt to prevent and to timely diagnose; (2) to facilitate, expedite, and enhance communication between people diagnosed and medical professionals; (3) to enable access to care for people living in remote areas (Farrell & McKinnon, 2003); and (4) to provide treatment in the form of various online therapies (Barak & Grohol, 2011; Ybarra & Eaton, 2005). Like in France, such tendencies were encouraged by the

---

[1] The other participating countries are the Netherlands (program leader), Belgium, Germany, Ireland, and the UK.

development of various strategies and pieces of legislation. For instance, already in 1996, the Electronic Freedom of Information Act (E-FOIA) Amendments mandated that governmental agencies provide information and make their records available in an electronic format (BIS, 2016; Department of Justice, 2014). Aware of people's increasing tendencies to look for information online, in May 2012, the White House launched the Digital Government Strategy, which aimed to further encourage agencies to use information and communication technologies (ICTs). It also provided guidance meant to assist them "to improve digital services and use emerging technologies to serve the public as effectively as possible" (OMB Memo 17-06, 2016). As a follow-up on this strategy, the White House released the U.S. Digital Service Playbook in 2014, which offered 13 main recommendations drawn from successful practices developed in the public as well as private sector (ibid.; The U.S. Digital Service, 2018). Despite such encouragement, agencies in both countries also encountered considerable challenges, as I will now discuss.

Technical Challenges: Accessibility Regulations for Online Platforms

While governmental agencies and mental healthcare providers were encouraged through political and legal measures to share their knowledge online, they also had to observe regulations concerning online accessibility. Worried that online information may not reach people with disabilities, in 1998 Section 508 of the Rehabilitation Act of 1973 was amended by the US Congress, requiring all Federal agencies "to make their electronic and information technology (EIT) accessible to people with disabilities" (Section 508.gov, 2017). Importantly, in January 2017, the US Access Board[2] ruled in favor of updating the requirements for ICTs mentioned under Section 508 and incorporated by reference the recommendations made by several voluntary consensus

---

[2] The US Access Board is a federal agency that aims to enhance the access of people with disabilities by providing guidelines and standards on various aspects, such as information technology, transportation, and medical equipment.

standards, such as those issued by the European Commission and the Web Content Accessibility Guidelines (WCAG 2.0). The latter are guidelines developed by the Web Accessibility Initiation (WAI) of the World Wide Web Consortium (W3C, 2017), which is the most important international standards organization for the Internet. This set of guidelines (WCAG 2.0), which became an ISO[3] standard in 2012, addresses new technologies and focuses not only on the accessibility of people with disabilities but also on that of people using more limiting devices, such as mobile phones rather than computers, laptops, or tablets. Building upon a European Parliament resolution from 2002,[4] similar legislation was passed in France in 2005. Article 47 of law no. 2005-102 of February 11, 2005 (Loi no. 2005-102), placed public agencies which shared information online under the obligation to render their websites accessible to people with disabilities. The recommendations inscribed in WCAG 2.0 were taken up in the third version of the Référentiel Géneral d'Accessibilité pour les Administrations (RGAA3), which defines the accessibility regulations that governmental agencies and public service providers in France are legally bound to observe. This document was updated in 2015 from RGAA 2.2, to which all French public websites were obliged to comply by May 2012.

According to WCAG 2.0, websites should be *perceivable, operable, understandable, and robust.* This means that the content put forward should be easy to see and hear and that any non-text content should be accompanied by text options, which can be more easily accessed using braille or speech, among others. At the same time, websites should be designed so that users can easily find their way around them, the information provided on them should be understandable, and the functions they contain should all be accessible using a keyboard. Furthermore, the content provided on websites should not cause seizures, and the compatibility of online platforms with "future user agents, including assistive technologies" should be enhanced (WCAG2.0). Governmental agencies and mental healthcare providers need therefore to make sure that the

---

[3] The International Organization for Standardization (ISO) is an international standard-setting body composed of representatives from various national standards organizations, which develops voluntary standards. In March 2017 ISO was working in 162 countries.

[4] The resolution is registered as COM (2001) 529–C5-0074/2002–2002/2032 (COS).

information they provide on their online platforms is accessible to people with different types of disabilities, to people with different levels of education, and to people whose modest income may mean that they cannot afford a computer, but can only look up such information using cheaper, less developed, or outdated technologies. While such requirements are necessary and laudable, it is important to note that they place significant constraints on these stakeholders regarding the ways in which they can use the Internet and the type of affordances they select for their websites.

Epistemic and Social Challenges: Critique of Psychiatry and Divergent Interests

While the accessibility requirement set upon governmental agencies and mental healthcare providers has led to challenges of a more technical nature, the public character of the Internet has contributed to some epistemic and social difficulties. This second set of challenges refers to the current context in which NIMH and HAS provide insights about bipolar disorder online, where the authority of such bodies is no longer readily accepted and their recommendations are not taken up without critical consideration. According to Rose, (2018:20), "[psychiatry's] very foundations came under attack from all sides" in the 1960s–1970s, and ever since, the expertise and authority of governmental agencies and mental healthcare providers has been challenged in various ways. Antipsychiatry emerged in that period as a movement which challenged the validity of psychiatric diagnostic and therapeutic practices, considering psychiatry to be an instrument of social oppression and control (Castel, 1976; Rose, 2018). Supporters of the movement further criticized the power imbalance at the heart of all forms of psychiatric treatments and the alienation of medical professionals from their patients. At the same time, many questioned the validity of psychiatric diagnoses, which they saw as arbitrary (McPherson & Armstrong, 2006; Wright & Cummings, 2005) and over-pathologizing (Horwitz & Wakefield, 2007; Scott, 2006), while others denounced the inhumane treatment of people placed in mental hospitals (Gostin, 2008; Morrison, 2013).

The degree to which such critics have opposed and continue to challenge psychiatry has varied as has their identity. Sometimes, criticism has been radical and has included, next to intellectuals, mental health professionals, with psychiatrists such as Szasz arguing that mental illness was a myth, a labeling mechanism through which the social and economic circumstances that dramatically affected people's lives were occluded from view (Szasz, 1961). Other mental health professionals such as Laing sought for a middle ground, founding residential homes and striving to develop more equal therapeutic approaches (Fussinger, 2011; Roberts & Itten, 2006). Similar variety has characterized the responses of people diagnosed, with some wholeheartedly embracing the medical model, with others arguing against specific medical interventions, such as forced containment and electroconvulsive therapy (ECT), and with yet others, ex-patients or self-entitled "survivors" of the mental health system (especially in the US) rejecting the medical model altogether (McLean, 2000).

Some authors (McLean, 2003; Rissmiller & Rissmiler, 2006) suggest that such antipsychiatric tendencies have been transformed and even integrated within the mental healthcare system they were once so critical of, in part due to psychiatry's reaction to the criticism received. Thus, psychiatry embraced a biomedical approach in efforts to render itself more scientific, a growing number of medical professionals started to value the insights of their patients, and the rights of the latter came to be codified in patient charters (Hopton, 2006). Furthermore, antipsychiatry supporters are claimed to have morphed in time into members of the broad consumer movement (McLean, 2003; Rissmiller & Rissmiler, 2006), which argues for the inclusion of people diagnosed in decision-making at all levels but which accepts the medical model of mental illness. Such stakeholders are satisfied with the fact that (in principle, at least) people diagnosed have the opportunity to choose the medical professionals they see and also have a say in the treatment they receive. According to proponents of such views, while more radical ex-patients/"survivors" still exist, a new type of consumer has come into being, who no longer shares the feelings of hopelessness of the ex-patients from the 1970s, nor the latter's strong criticism and suspicion toward mental healthcare professionals.

An overview of books and articles published in the last two decades suggests, however, that such claims about the successful rapprochement between former antipsychiatry supporters and medical institutions underestimate the critical atmosphere which continues to surround psychiatry. Numerous psychiatrists remain critical of their specialty and have come together in various organizations, such as *The International Critical Psychiatry Network*, to exchange views and to seek to develop alternatives to the current dominant approach. At the same time, they call for drastic reform of the mental healthcare system, arguing that accessibility and quality of care remain importantly dependent on markers of identity, such as class, race, and gender (Hopton, 2006; Metzl, 2009). Another group of critics accuses current psychiatry of medicalization or imperialistic tendencies, as normal aspects of life and behavior, such as mourning, have become pathologized (Lane, 2009). While some commentators consider psychiatry as a political science since its very inception (Rose, 2018), others see an augmentation of its politicization and argue that it puts forward views that have little scientific backing in order to serve particular interests and to uphold certain social values (Wright & Cummings, 2005). Yet others decry the medicalization of mental health conditions in that it focuses solely on medications and neglects social provisions, which are highly necessary for the recovery and social reintegration of people diagnosed (Kinderman, 2014).

Psychiatrists and journalists alike have criticized the close relation between psychiatrists and pharmaceutical companies (Carlat, 2010; Kirsch, 2010; Whitaker, 2010). From this point of view, some deplore the fact that most research on the effectiveness of specific medications is conducted by the pharmaceutical companies themselves, which suggests the results may be biased (Whitaker, 2010). Others downright challenge the effectiveness of medical treatments, arguing, for instance, that there is no significant difference between the effects of antidepressants and those of placebo (Kirsch & Sapirstein, 1998). There are also voices who warn that the promotion of self-determination and empowerment of people diagnosed with mental health conditions may be superficial and represent a political move rather than genuine interest and appreciation for their insights (Bernstein, 2006; Hopton, 2006). A staunch opponent of psychiatry remains the *Church of Scientology*, which funds the *Citizens*

Commission on Human Rights, the museum *Psychiatry: Industry of Death*, and which disseminates various materials harshly criticizing the effects of psychotropic drugs as well as the motives and intentions of this profession.

Apart from medical professionals, sociologists, and journalists, critical psychiatric tendencies continue to be put forward by people diagnosed. From this point of view, the Internet has enabled many opponents to come together. According to Whitley (2012:1040), "[t]he Internet has given a means for current and former psychiatric patients, who sometimes refer to themselves as 'survivors', to widely disseminate often negative attitudes, beliefs, experiences, and opinions vis-a-vis psychiatry." An example is *The Antipsychiatry Coalition*, an organization which aims "to warn you of the harm routinely inflicted on those who receive psychiatric 'treatment' and to promote the democratic ideal of liberty for all law-abiding people" at an international level. They challenge the medical understanding of mental health conditions and the scientific bases for the medical treatment prescribed, accusing it to be "quackery," and organize various actions to raise awareness, such as the Electroshock Protest, which took place on May 16, 2015, in the US. Highly influential in this sense is also Monica Cassani's blog, *Beyond Meds*. An ex-patient and mental health professional, Cassani claims that this dual position enables her to share "some interesting and sometimes uncomfortable insights into the mental health system in the United States" (Cassani, 2017). Other ex-patients continue to refuse the medical model of mental illness, arguing instead that their experiences represent different ways of being in the world, and such views are promoted by groups such as the *Hearing Voices Network* (Hopton, 2006; Romme & Escher, 1993).

The various types of critique enumerated above indicate that there continue to be important differences even among mental health professionals regarding their understanding and approach to mental health. Such differences of opinion are augmented by the various reforms which have been brought to the mental healthcare system in the US and France (Hochmann, 2017), as by limiting insurance coverage and the number of (prospective) specialists, these reforms have led to the marginalization of previously successful professionals, such as psychoanalysts in France (Pignarre, 2006). At the same time, different types of mental healthcare professionals often find themselves in competition for limited resources or have to take over functions and tasks previously fulfilled by other specialists (Desmettre, 2009; Gill et al., 2014). Furthermore, this also seems to prompt some of them to embrace divergent interests and to advocate different approaches. Psychologists often reduce psychiatry to the mere provision of medical treatment and accuse it of neglecting the full person of the person diagnosed. Furthermore, by focusing too much on genetic and neurological factors, psychologists and social therapists argue that important environmental factors are neglected. To the accusation that they merely prescribe psychotropic drugs, psychiatrists reply by pointing to general practitioners as the professionals who often prescribe higher dosages and more medicines than they recommend. As a reaction to extreme biomedicalization, psychoanalysts seem to be making a comeback in the US, even though access to them is heavily restricted by insurance policies (Chessick, 2006; Maness, 2017; O'Sullivan, 2016). In France, the conflict between psychoanalysts and psychiatrists is still fresh (Pignarre, 2006). For instance, a report from 2009 for the Minister of Health and Sports, Roselyne Bachelot, where three approaches to mental health were evaluated, caused a lot of uproar. At a more general level, mental healthcare providers decry the influence of managed care controls and the cost containment policies which have been taken up over the last few decades, and which severely reduce their autonomy and ability to make treatment decisions freely (Scheid, 2000). It is in this context, fraught by different types of challenges, that the online provision of information about bipolar disorder by governmental agencies and mental healthcare providers takes place. Succeeding to perform expertise about bipolar disorder online in such circumstances becomes a rather remarkable feat, which needs to be carefully studied.

Rhetoric and the Performance of Expertise Online

In the field of STS, there is a rich tradition of studies on the construction of scientific knowledge (Bijker et al., 2009; Knorr Cetina, 1999; MacKenzie, 1990; Shapin & Schaffer, 1985/2011), whereby the importance of social, political, and economic factors in processes which for a long time have been claimed to be neutral has been highlighted. In this sense, Felt remarked that "[m]aking knowledge is …never an 'innocent' activity; nothing can be regarded as 'natural' or 'simply given'" (Felt, 2017:253). Important to understand the work that goes into the construction of scientific facts is the work of Latour (1987), who shows that "science in the making" is messy, subject to heated debates and controversies, which are often solved by making strategic alliances or by using one's social capital (Bourdieu, 1975). In what follows, I will discuss how governmental agencies perform expertise about bipolar disorder online, which means that I will not focus on the construction of scientific facts, but will trace, instead, the manners in which they are made available online, their unfolding destiny on these platforms. For this purpose, I adjust the notion of performance put forward by Goffman (1959/1990) building upon insights acquired from its application in the study of scientific authority (Hilgartner, 2000) and the suggestion that this concept may be amenable to the investigation of phenomena involving digital technologies (Hafermalz et al., 2016). Performance thus (re)conceived was combined with insights from Latour on the rhetorical techniques through which scientific facts are constructed and with perspectives from media studies (Drucker, 2011) on the role of various web interface elements on users' experiences. This innovative approach allowed for various digital objects and technologies to be approached as actors fulfilling different roles and functions in the performance of the two institutions studied here, and focused the analysis on the ways in which seemingly disparate elements—aesthetic, functional, content-related—were combined to put forward specific perspectives on bipolar disorder for particular audiences.

Rhetoric plays an important role in the complex trajectory statements that follow from mere hypotheses or "hunches" to scientific facts (Latour, 1987; Latour & Woolgar, 1979). It also lends itself to the analysis of the relations between the different types of knowledge used in mental healthcare, as positive or negative modalities, which imbue statements with lower or greater degrees of certainty, can convey the dominance of particular ways of understanding while subtly discarding or diminishing others. Such rhetorical techniques are integral part of a performance, but their effects are shaped by other important elements: *the team and team-mates,* who put up the performance, and who can take up different roles, that is, director, actors; *the setting,* that is the environment where the performance takes place; *sign equipment* consisting of various props that help foster the impression intended by the performance; and *the audi-ence,* consisting of those for whom the performance is put up (Goffman, 1990/1959). Whereas the sign equipment and stage Goffman had in mind were of a different material character, the choice of web design elements, the visual cues provided contribute to the production of meaning on online platforms (Drucker, 2013). I therefore suggest that the online technologies these institutions use and the online practices they engage in help foreground particular insights about bipolar disorder while downplaying others. This has implications not only for how this condition is understood by online readers, but also for the credibility and standing of NIMH and HAS.

Important for the success of a performance is the division of the stage into two regions—the front and backstage—which can be accessed by different people and where different behaviors can be taken up. Whereas the frontstage refers to the totality of actions and props that the actors engage with and use in their performance that are visible to the audience, the backstage refers to the elements that one needs to occlude from view in order to guarantee a successful performance, information to which the audience's access is purposefully impeded. The comparison of the information on bipolar disorder made available online by NIMH and HAS at different moments in time allowed for the identification of novel elements entering the frontstage as well as of insights and perspectives which were downplayed or given up upon. I therefore suggest that in the case of online performances, there may be two types of backstage worth considering: the "conventional" one that Goffman (1959/1990) described, containing interactions and negotiations among the online platform developers, debates among scientists, drafts of the information intended to be made available, and the tools and technologies used for these activities; and a "digital" backstage, containing older versions of the performance and revealing the affordances previously available on these platforms. By comparing them with the current performance, elements which NIMH and HAS may seek to conceal are unearthed. Whereas access to the first type of backstage was not possible for the study described here, the "digital" backstage could be visited by collecting and comparing data from the online platforms at three different moments in time. Data used in this analysis consist therefore of the online pages dedicated to bipolar disorder on the website of NIMH and HAS, and they were collected in 2014, 2015, and 2016.

The success of a performance does not only depend on the talent of the actors and the quality of their parts, but it is also importantly shaped by the stage decorum. Insights from media studies reveal that elements of visual design importantly shape the meaning of the information made available on an online platform. Thus, the quantity of information provided on a particular aspect, where the information is placed on a website, the font size and type, how the information is visually framed by banners and advertisements, a dynamic or static environment, and the type and position of the menu as well as the writing style used guide readers toward particular bits of information, and help them distinguish important insights from less relevant ones (Moshagen & Thielsch, 2010). The use of color is also very important, as color patterns help readers recognize how information is structured and organized; the contrast between foreground and background importantly affects a website's readability, while the number and kind of colors used and their distribution on the website affect readers' ability to concentrate and may imbue the information with particular connotations (Cyr & Trevor-Smith, 2004; Flemming, 1998). Next to these elements, the navigability of an online platform and the affordances available to their users importantly shape users' attitude toward the insights provided. Given the important role they play in the production of meaning and the great variety of ways in which they can be combined online, these elements were also considered when analyzing how NIMH and HAS perform expertise about bipolar disorder online. The data collected and analyzed consist therefore of texts, videos, images, and hyperlinks. In the following, I describe the main performative techniques identified and present images and extracts to illustrate the approaches and online elements that helped put forward particular understandings of bipolar disorder.

Performative Techniques and Online Expertise About Bipolar Disorder

NIMH and the Quest for the Redefinition of Bipolar Disorder

NIMH is the main agency of the American government responsible for biomedical and health-related research. It is the largest research organization in the world focusing on mental health. With a budget of about $1.5 billion, NIMH conducts its own research, but also largely determines the national research agenda by providing grants to other institutes and organizations throughout the US. In what may be seen as an attempt to counter anti-psychiatric tendencies, since the 1980s, NIMH has also started to pay more attention to the perspectives and insights of people diagnosed with mental health conditions. For instance, it has funded self-help agencies managed by former patients or self-titled "consumers," which nowadays together constitute *The Center for Mental Health Services*. At the same time, NIMH has launched two research centers with the task to study the activity of self-help groups and the (therapeutic) effectiveness of such initiatives among people diagnosed with severe mental health conditions (Borkman, 1997). Important to understand the highly influential position NIMH occupies is the distinction between being "in authority" and being "an authority" put forward by Jongen (2017). Being *in* authority refers to the mandate certain governmental bodies receive to develop rules and regulations and even to make decisions for others. Being *an* authority is linked to the epistemic authority of certain institutions or people, and highlights the relation between the bearers of such authority and those who grant it. NIMH is therefore both in authority, by actively shaping the activities of numerous institutions and self-help groups, and an authority because of the prestige it enjoys. Furthermore, it is endowed with sufficient resources to shape its online presence as its representatives best see it fit.

By analyzing the online materials described above, I found that NIMH performed expertise about bipolar disorder online as stable and authoritative and achieved this by prioritizing on its platform understandings and approaches that could lend themselves more easily to observable and quantifiable investigations. Important in this sense was the understanding of bipolar disorder that NIMH put forward. Whereas this condition is generally conceived as a "mood disorder" and the role of the brain in its onset and development is still debated, NIMH referred to the brain being its main causal factor as an unproblematic fact. According to the institute (2014, 2015, 2016), "[b]ipolar disorder, also known as manic-depressive illness, is a brain disorder that causes unusual shifts in mood, energy, activity levels, and the ability to carry out day-to-day tasks."

This seemingly stable and unproblematic definition of bipolar disorder was maintained through the deployment of three sets of omissions and by operating an important modification to a related concept. Thus, while bipolar disorder was defined rather unproblematically as a brain condition throughout the time period studied, the definition of a mood episode was broadened to include next to emotional states (2014) also different levels of energy and types of behavior (2016). Thus, NIMH modified the weight ascribed to the various markers of this condition and, in so doing, put forward a more complex image of bipolar disorder. This challenges the views of commentators who have expressed concern that the rise of "the brain" in mental health research would oversimplify how mental health conditions are understood and approached. The fact that moods were brought by NMH on a par with other aspects, such as one's ability to engage in various acts, does foreground, however, more quantifiable approaches to how bipolar disorder is diagnosed, as medical professionals need to assess a person's behaviors along a growing number of dimensions and at a more granular level. Thus, whereas the definition of bipolar disorder seemingly stayed the same, the means by which this condition can be known were transformed. Bipolar disorder thus gradually became a condition which can be more easily recognized and monitored from the outside, even in the absence of highly deviant behaviors, and, importantly given the various digital and AI-based technologies discussed in the first chapter, along quantifiable markers.

Despite this important change, NIMH succeeded to perform expertise about bipolar disorder as stable and unproblematic by operating three sets of omissions: (1) keeping backstage insights about its changing perspective on bipolar disorder; (2) not providing information on how scientific, social, and technological factors inform this perspective; and (3) not engaging with its societal significance. These omissions were successfully achieved through a shrewd combination of rhetoric and the use of specific sign equipment, that is, of specific digital affordances. Thus, the impression of epistemic stability was supported by NIMH's decision to dress its main character in the modest costume of digital text, which gives the illusion of permanence and immutability. No further details were given regarding the designer(s) of this costume, when it was produced and how. Building upon Latour's (1987) insights, this choice may have been informed by NIMH's desire to highlight the scientific character of the information it provided, by rendering it "devoid of any trace of ownership, construction, time and place" (Latour, 1987:23). Yet, a look into the backstage of NIMH's platform, that is, at records of the information previously available on its main page dedicated to bipolar disorder, revealed that in 2014 the institute was more optimistic about the genetic causes of this condition, both in terms of content and the amount of space dedicated to them:

> Bipolar disorder tends to run in families. Some research has suggested that people with certain genes are more likely to develop bipolar disorder than others. Children with a parent or sibling who has bipolar disorder are much more likely to develop the illness, compared with children who do not have a family history of bipolar disorder. However, most children with a family history of bipolar disorder will not develop the illness. (…) But genes are not the only risk factor for bipolar disorder. Studies of identical twins have shown that the twin of a person with bipolar illness does not always develop the disorder, despite the fact that identical twins share all of the same genes. (NIMH, 2014)

Whereas in 2014, NIMH did not hesitate to suggest bipolar disorder may be a condition occurring in families, by 2016 the language it used about genetic causes had become more tentative:

> Some research suggests that people with certain genes are more likely to develop bipolar disorder than others. But genes are not the only risk factor for bipolar disorder. Studies of identical twins have shown that even if one twin develops bipolar disorder, the other twin does not always develop the

disorder, despite the fact that identical twins share all of the same genes. (NIMH, 2016)

The 2016 text may be seen as an attempt to preempt alarm among the relatives of people diagnosed with bipolar disorder, and its brevity suggests that NIMH may have assumed this information not to be particularly interesting for its audience. The use of indefinite adverbs and adjectives, such as "some" and "certain," and the omission of any references does not encourage the audience to look further into these matters. The audience is therefore expected to believe these statements simply because they have been uttered by a stakeholder already recognized as an authority. While it makes sense to retain on the website the most up-to-date insights about bipolar disorder, this comparison highlights the performative effects of the "presentism" that digital platforms afford, particularly when the focus can be maintained on the frontstage. Thus, the possibility to avoid any discussion of the processes and evaluations whereby content is modified helped promote an image of NIMH's expertise about bipolar disorder as stable and unquestionable.

This impression of stability was also reinforced by NIMH's omitting of any insights about the factors that influence its orientation as to the most fruitful areas of research into the causes of bipolar disorder. Whereas describing bipolar disorder as a brain condition favors a neuroscientific approach to it, NIMH did not share any details regarding the type and amount of scientific evidence which led it to support this conceptualization. Nor did it indicate to what extent advances in neuroimaging technologies and techniques prompted it to consider that "the brains of people with bipolar disorder may differ from the brains of healthy people or people with other mental disorders" (NIMH, 2017). In so doing, NIMH occluded from the audience's view the role factors such as the dynamic assessments of scientific feasibility, the changing popularity and influence of specific scientific fields, charismatic scientists, available technologies, financial costs, and administrative and organizational obstacles play in such processes of knowledge production.

NIMH further omitted to publicly consider the societal significance of its conceptualization, to ponder on how the understanding of bipolar disorder as a "brain condition" that can be measured and monitored along numerous parameters may impact on the types of mental health professionals involved and on the work they do, on the experiences of people diagnosed with this condition, and on the social provisions they are entitled to. Through such omissions, the institute positioned this knowledge as natural, obvious, unproblematic. In so doing, I argue that NIMH performed yet another type of omission, as it appeared rather oblivious to the distrust some people experience in regard to psychiatry and governmental institutions, discussed in the earlier sections of this chapter. All these are issues that NIMH kept backstage, successfully occluding them from view in its performance.

The Role of Sign Equipment in NIMH's Performance on Bipolar Disorder

As already mentioned in the previous chapter, the type of platform a particular stakeholder chooses depends on its status, on the resources it has available, and on its goals. From a financial and technical point of view, non-interactive online platforms are less challenging, as they represent variations upon options which have been available since the early days of the Internet. Considering the relatively simple technologies and programming functions required for their development as well as their limited interactive potential, non-interactive online platforms may be seen as rather conservative options in the current digital environment. They are hardly ideal for governmental agencies which aim to educate their audiences and encourage them to use (certified) online resources. Furthermore, in a context where such official bodies find themselves under the obligation to have an online presence, opting for a non-interactive online platform does not help them position themselves as open and transparent. Nevertheless, such platforms continue to be the preferred choice for many official institutions, which seem to be more interested in making information available to the public rather than also acquiring direct insights into the public's views and experiences.

NIMH opted for a non-interactive online platform, and its considerable budget suggests that this choice was motivated by other reasons than financial concerns. If we look at the information NIMH provided on its online platform as a performance, then the visual, structural, and functional aspects of the site (see Fig. 3.1) represent important elements of the sign equipment used, which are meant to contribute to a persuasive performance. The ways in which information is structured and organized on the platform together with the choices that were made regarding webpage and navigation design are relevant, because they help orient the audience toward particular understandings (Djonov, 2007).

As can be seen in Fig. 3.1,[5] NIMH opted for a rather minimalist visual design for its online platform. Blue and gray were the main colors used and they fulfilled important functions, as they highlighted specific rubrics or content. The choice of colors is in line with the WCAG 2.0 recommendations, which mention that a good distinction between foreground and background enhances readability. By choosing to give its performance in a minimalist *setting*, I argue that NIMH revealed its awareness of the highly authoritative position it occupies, of the fact that it does not need to use any apparent embellishments to draw crowds in for its performance. Furthermore, this apparent simplicity may fulfill another important rhetoric function, as it might signal to the audience that the scope of the performance is to reveal the truth about bipolar disorder without any artifice and in an unbiased fashion. The sober colors used on the platform together with the basic affordances can thus be interpreted as a visual enactment of scientific rigor and authority. At the same time, they also steer the audience to focus on the content made available.

While the visual design of the site is how NIMH chose to decorate the stage for its performance, I consider the platform's rubrics to be *stage props*, which contributed to the institution's self-presentation and revealed the targeted audience and the type of relation NIMH envisaged with it. Thus, the information it made available about bipolar disorder was placed under the more general rubric entitled "Health & Education," which indicated that the insights provided were meant for the general population and not for mental healthcare professionals. In so doing, NIMH seemed to be positively responding to the various measures taken by US

---

[5] For more information on some sign equipment elements and an overview of the specific roles they play in NIMH's performance, see Table 2.2 in the Appendix. The red numbers in these images were added by the author for analytic purposes.

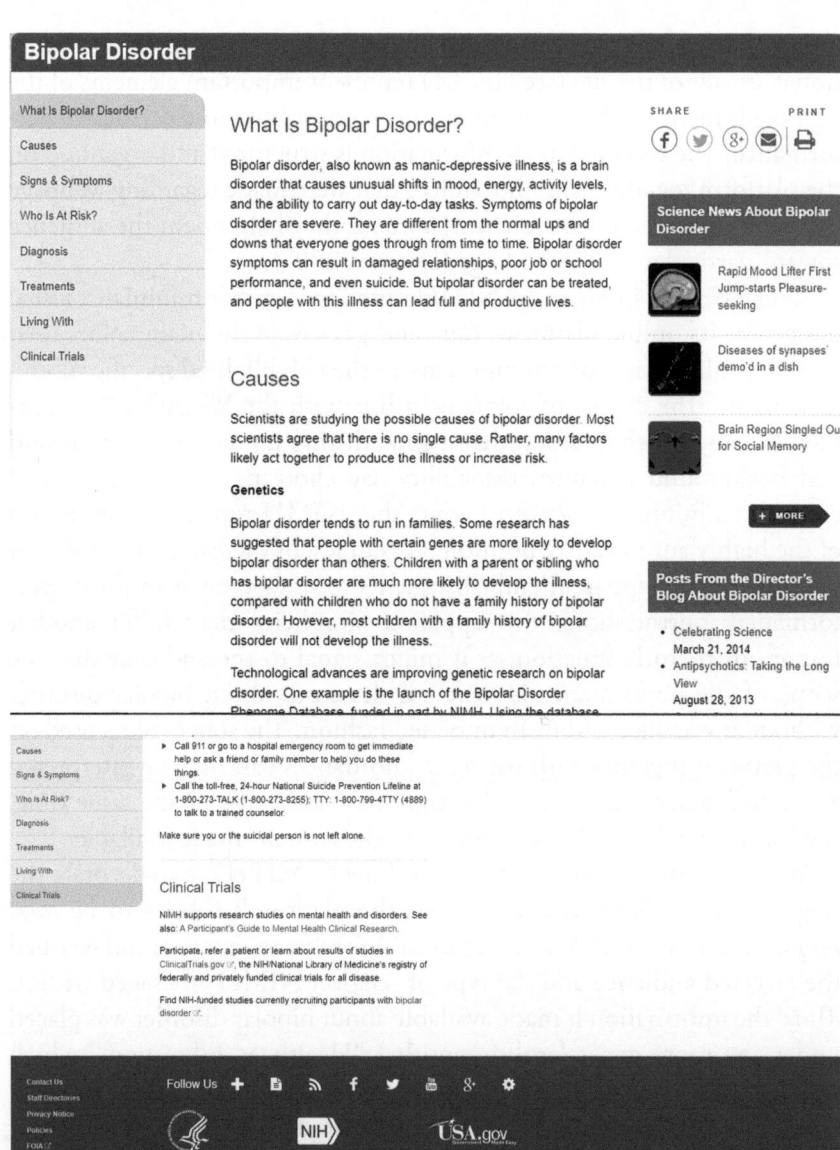

Fig. 3.1 Images of the upper and lower parts of NIMH's website (2016)

authorities to encourage the use of the Internet for mental health-related education. The horizontal rubrics at the top—mental health information; statistics; consumer health publications; help for mental illnesses; clinical trials—brought together different types of knowledge and positioned NIMH as an institution devoted to furthering scientific knowledge while being appreciative of the insights shared by people diagnosed with mental health conditions. At the same time, these rubrics helped remind the audience that the institute is dedicated not only to research but also to improving the lives of people diagnosed.

Whereas the rubrics at the top of the website served self-presentation purposes and focused on the institute's missions and prerogatives, those in the lower part of the page revealed how it used its online platform. Thus, they contained brief clarifications regarding NIMH's position on FOIA, accessibility, privacy, its policies, and the ways in which it could be contacted. Regarding accessibility, NIMH assured its readers that it "is making every effort to ensure that the information available on our website is accessible to all. To meet this commitment, we have designed our site to comply with Section 508 of the Rehabilitation Act." Nevertheless, NIMH reserved for itself the right to decide how to fulfill this commitment. Thus, while the static character of its website facilitated its accessibility, it did not provide text alternatives for some of the videos put up. From this point of view, it would appear that NIMH used the accessibility guidelines in ways which allowed it to opt for the platform design and online affordances that it preferred.

Important insights regarding the goals of the performance NIMH put up and about its intended audience were provided under the rubric "Policies," where it became apparent that the institute mainly focused on the general public rather than medical professionals. In so doing, NIMH was wary not to jeopardize or diminish the authority and prerogatives of medical professionals, as it

> does not intend to provide specific medical advice on our Web sites, but rather to help visitors better understand mental health and disorders. NIMH will not provide specific medical advice and urges you to consult with a qualified mental health or health care provider for diagnosis and for answers to your personal questions.

In line with the institute's penchant for conservative choices regarding its online platform, the role of the audience to the performance was limited. It could not engage in processes of knowledge production and evaluation through direct reactions, nor could it publicly challenge in this online space the vision of bipolar disorder NIMH put up. Furthermore, the peripheral position ascribed to the option "Contact Us" suggested that dealing with public inquiries was not a function NIMH prioritized. While localized engagement or resistance was this way discouraged, the audience was allowed, however, to play an active role in ensuring the circulation of NIMH's insights by printing, e-mailing, or sharing them on social media. Even though these online affordances are common elements on most websites nowadays, I argue that they fulfilled a performative function nonetheless, as they suggested that the knowledge NIMH made available was relevant and interesting enough for people to want to keep it or to inform others about.

The simplicity and clarity of the platform was aligned with the ways in which the part of the main actor was structured and worded. Thus, NIMH's perspective on bipolar disorder was organized along the following rubrics: definition; signs and symptoms; risk factors; treatments and therapies; join a study; and learn more. As these rubrics already suggest, the information provided contributed to a performance whereby bipolar disorder was presented as a complex but manageable condition. A hopeful, optimistic tone was maintained by mentioning ongoing studies meant to shed further light on its causes and reveal fruitful new forms of treatment. The vertically organized rubrics on the right played an important role in supporting this perspective, as they helped convey a dynamic, productive view on bipolar disorder research, with new insights being frequently put forward and new studies developed for people to join. The mobile character of these videos and hyperlinks had a double function, as they helped highlight the stability and importance of the main actor, and also reminded the audience of NIMH's prerogative and dedication to tackle the complexity of bipolar disorder. Thus, whereas the institute was rather conservative in how it performed expertise, it did use the latest approaches to online technologies when they served its purposes.

Goffman's dramaturgical approach helped highlight some specific ways in which the (visual) design of NIMH's online platform and the online affordances available on it participated in shaping the meaning of bipolar disorder and the institute's public image. Sharing information online requires important coordination work between distinct elements and the choice of these elements is often indicative of the type of audience targeted and how it is expected to engage with the information provided, as the discussion of HAS' performative techniques will indicate.

HAS' Performative Techniques to Redefine Bipolar Disorder

HAS is an independent public institution with a scientific character, created in 2004. Its board consists of eight members appointed for six years (with the possibility of renewal every three years) by the President of France (two members can be proposed by the President, two by the President of the Senate, two by the President of the National Assembly, and two by the President of the Economic, Social, and Environmental Council (CESE)). HAS fulfills three main functions: (i) to evaluate from a medical and economic point of view health products, technologies, and practices in view of their admission for reimbursement (a French version of Health Technology Assessment); (ii) to provide recommendations on healthcare practices and public health; to create guide books on treatment for patients and medical professionals; to develop medico-economic studies; to advise public institutions in their decisions regarding public health, and to define the trajectory of personalized care to which one is entitled; and (iii) to certify healthcare establishments and to provide accreditations for medical professionals. Very important for this study is that HAS also certifies health-related online platforms. Its current annual budget is €60 million, and its revenue comes from taxes on promotional spending by drug companies, National Health Insurance, state funding, HONcode accreditation fees, payment for assessing applications for inclusion on reimbursement lists, and so on.

Based on the online materials examined, I found that HAS performed expertise about bipolar disorder online so as to assist in the reform of the French mental healthcare system. As mentioned in the previous chapter, France struggles due to an insufficient number of psychiatrists, and one of the solutions that have been put forward in recent years has been to more extensively involve other medical professionals in the provision of mental healthcare. General practitioners (GPs) are among those meant to take over some of the responsibilities previously bestowed upon psychiatrists. To better prepare the GPs, HAS provided them with important and varied insights and thereby made ample use of the fact that the architecture of online platforms rendered the existence of multiple simultaneous frontstages possible. The agency thus developed three frontstages where it put up different but related performances about bipolar disorder: a memo card with recommended practices for the diagnostic and management of bipolar disorder (2015); a press communication in HAS' online magazine (2015); and a guide for bipolar disorder as a chronic condition (2016) (Fig. 3.3). In so doing, HAS indicated its awareness that it was in authority to provide its intended audience of medical professionals with guidelines regarding various tasks and competencies, ranging from the correct diagnosis of bipolar disorder, to familiarity with the new distribution of duties and responsibilities between GPs, psychiatrists, other mental healthcare professionals, and patients (see Figs. 3.2 and 3.3), to indications of the types of therapeutic interventions that were officially reimbursed (see Fig. 3.3). This way, HAS performed expertise about bipolar disorder through the provision of recommendations regarding diagnostic and therapeutic practices and a clear distribution of responsibilities. In what follows I will zoom into its performance of expertise through the memo card and will show that unlike NIMH, which made efforts to steer away from dramatic overtones and to maintain the impression of stability in regard to its perspective on bipolar disorder, HAS actively engaged in the reconceptualization of this condition by operating several plot twists.

This performance took place on a stage where three main actors shared information (see Fig. 3.2): (1) a storyteller that informed the public about the aims with which HAS had developed the memo card and the audience it addressed; (2) a main character, the memo card, which consisted of an overview of practices meant to help doctors diagnose and treat bipolar disorder efficiently and effectively; and (3) another main character, the report on the elaboration of the memo card, which effectively transported the audience backstage, revealing the processes and

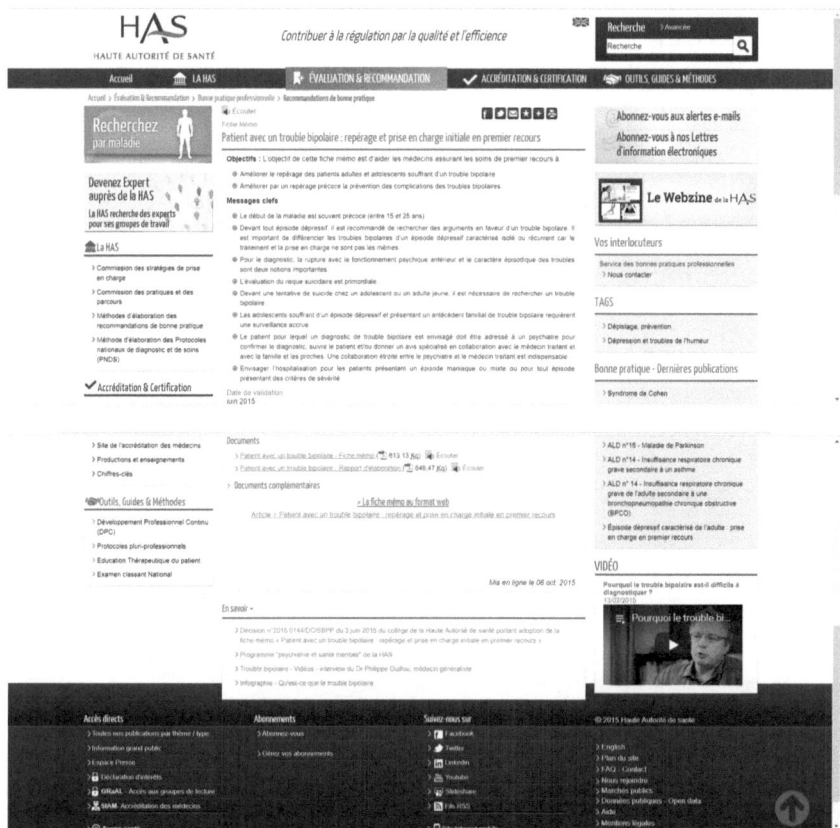

Fig. 3.2   Images of the upper and lower parts of HAS' online page on the diagnostic and treatment of bipolar disorder

negotiations through which the memo card came into being. Whereas NIMH understood bipolar disorder as a brain condition, HAS focused on its "evolution" in time and reconstructed bipolar disorder as a largely developmental or degenerative condition. The agency stated, for instance, that the periods of remission between episodes would get shorter in time, especially if bipolar disorder was not treated, whereas the number of depressive episodes would become more frequent and last longer. HAS thus emphasized the importance of correctly diagnosing this condition as early as possible, it signaled its severity, and it highlighted the relevance of

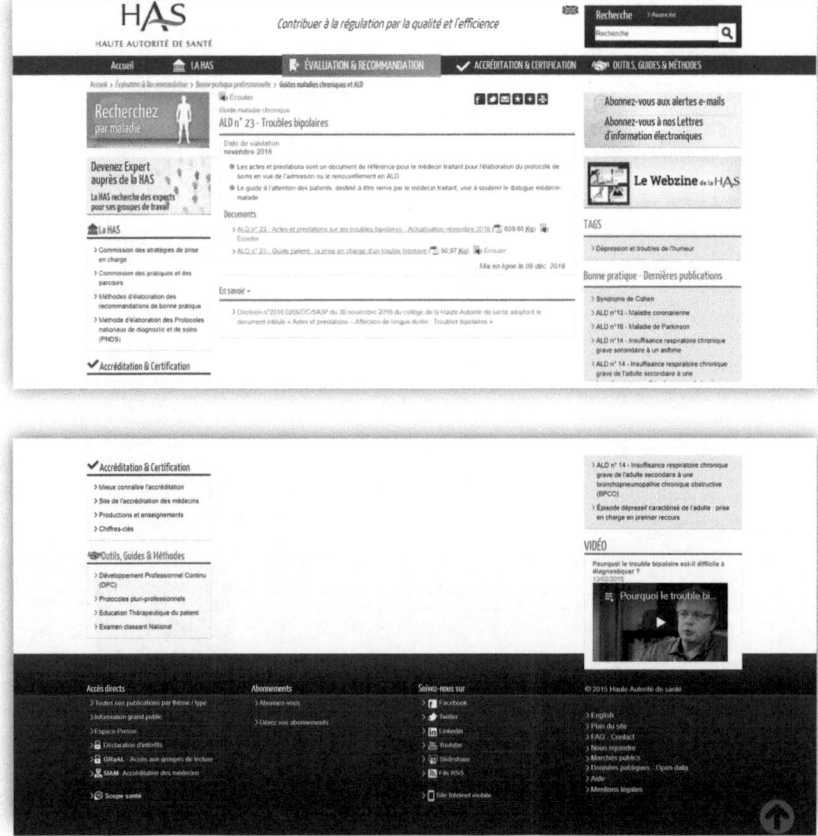

Fig. 3.3 Images of the upper and lower parts of HAS' online page dedicated to bipolar disorder as a chronic condition

treatment. Since it also heightened the pressure for medical professionals to correctly identify bipolar disorder, such a redefinition functioned as a performative technique through which HAS sought to achieve one of its stated goals, namely the reduction of diagnostic delay (HAS, 2015a).

To this aim, HAS further operated another and, arguably, most dramatic twist in its performance of expertise about bipolar disorder, as it depicted suicidal attempts as symptoms of this condition and described bipolar disorder as "a highly suicidogenic pathology" (2016). Since statistics confer an aura of objectivity and credibility to the information provided, making it seem more factual and more urgent (Potter, 1996), the main actor called upon them, to legitimate this understanding of bipolar disorder. Thus, it warned the audience that one out of two people diagnosed with this condition would make at least one suicide attempt and that at least one out of ten untreated patients would commit suicide, which accounted for 15% of the population of people diagnosed with bipolar disorder. The performance HAS put up on this frontstage was aligned with its institutional role, as through it, the agency guided medical professionals in the assessment of the suicide risk their patients posed. It did so by developing indicators specific to bipolar disorder: an early onset of the condition; the presence of mixed characteristics; rapid cycles; the presence of psychotic symptoms; alcohol addiction; and addiction to illicit substances or to other psychoactive substances. Furthermore, HAS engaged in the construction of new categories, as it put forward a specific assessment of a suicidal crisis—low, medium, high—and positioned social isolation as an indicator of medium or high level. In so doing, the agency framed the ability to assess the risk of suicide as one of the competencies that medical professionals involved in the management of this condition needed to master. The attention to the new skills and abilities required marks an important difference between HAS and NIMH, as the latter omitted to include in its performance of expertise considerations about the ways in which changes in its understanding and approach to bipolar disorder would shape the work of medical professionals.

The presence of the report on the elaboration of the memo card as another main actor of this frontstage illustrates HAS' commitment to transparency and public accountability. This document indicated the credentials of the team of experts involved, testified to the depth and breadth of the literature reviewed, and revealed the numerous actors that were consulted before the final product—the memo card—was publicly made available: different types of medical professionals, several patient organizations, non-governmental organizations, etc. It thus rendered transparent the processes by which the memo card came into being and transported the audience onto the backstage. Whereas such information was absent from the online platform of NIMH, possibly in order to avoid any liability and potential causes for litigation, the audience of HAS had thus the opportunity to understand the tremendous scientific and diplomatic effort involved in such an undertaking, and was invited to appreciate this institution's inclusive character. By placing on the frontstage a document which one generally expects to find relegated to the backstage, HAS sought to legitimate and heighten the acceptability and authority of the memo card, while also positioning itself as a reliable, transparent, and democratic institution.

The Role of Sign Equipment in HAS' Performance of Expertise

The structure of the performance HAS put up and its choice of stage equipment were by no means accidental, but were aligned with the intended audience and educational purposes. HAS' performance was organized as a series of monologues, with each individual character taking its turn to play its part. The main characters were dressed in the simple and conservative outfit of portable document format (pdf) files, whereas some of the side actors were wrapped in the equally conservative suit of digital text. These choices enabled the audience to focus upon what each character had to say without any interruptions, contradictions, or divagations. At the same time, by wearing such hard and impenetrable costumes, each part the characters had to say, every insight and practical advice about bipolar disorder that they provided acquired stability and authority, which befit scientific facts. Furthermore, pdf files allow for relevant information to be highlighted and easily identified, they enable users to add their own thoughts and ideas in the form of comments and notes, and they can be accessed from a variety of devices. Thus, not only did such attires allow HAS to fulfill the WCAG 2.0 accessibility recommendations, but they could also be more readily consumed by careful and goal-oriented readers, such as treating doctors, who need to act quickly and who require stability and coherence in their practices.

The doctors' projected increase in workload and the need for efficiency may have prompted HAS to endow some of its main actors with an additional costume, the audio file. The audience could thus have a say in how these actors brought forward their monologues, as it could listen, read, or opt for a combination of the two. Furthermore, the audience could also take in the performance with the additional help of a "reading ruler,"

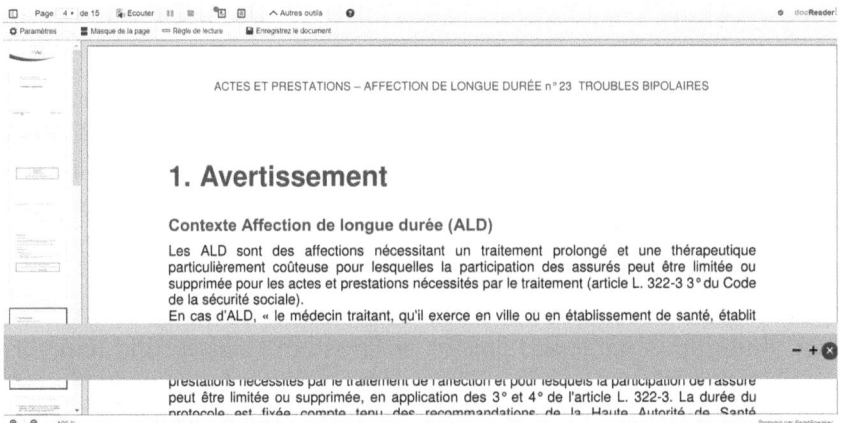

Fig. 3.4 Image of the affordances—audio and reading ruler—of a .pdf file provided by HAS

which allowed it to read in a more focused way or to keep up with the pace of the speaker (Fig. 3.4). This way, HAS made it possible for treating doctors to choose a format which was better aligned with their personal studying or memorizing techniques, as some would focus better using visual means and others audio props, while yet others a combination thereof. Furthermore, while the typed text required the audience to focus mainly upon it, the audio format enabled it to also listen to HAS' advice when engaged in other activities.

As the distribution of roles and the choice of decorum indicate, HAS staged its performance on bipolar disorder as a rather idyllic world, where the best results could be achieved when treating doctors corroborate their treatment decisions with legal provisions regarding the insurance and reimbursement of medical care and when they provide their patients with documentation meant "to support the dialogue" between them. Given the currently fraught relations between different types of mental health professionals in France, this approach may have been taken in order to provide an example for its medical audiences to follow, as an attempt to achieve not only informational but also behavioral changes. These considerations may have therefore informed HAS' choice of costume for its characters as well as the way in which it organized the reverberations of several plot twists across different regions of its three stages.

Discussion

This chapter discussed the performative techniques through which two highly influential institutions performed expertise about bipolar disorder online, in a context in which official bodies are required to make their insights available via the Internet, but face important challenges to their authority, and need to respect specific technical provisions. It showed that NIMH and HAS performed expertise about bipolar disorder in different ways, as NIMH used various strategies to depict its perspective on this condition as stable and precise, whereas HAS actively and transparently engaged in its redefinition to assist in the reform of the French mental healthcare. The type of information shared depended on the intended audience, and the visual design and most of the affordances available on the online platforms of these institutions helped the audience better find their way while reiterating the authoritative position of NIMH and HAS. As we have seen, these institutions were not enthusiastic users of the Internet, exploring its full potential and experimenting with the latest online technologies. Instead, they opted for non-interactive online platforms, reminiscent of the Web 1.0 era, with static content and limited interactivity. Combined with various rhetorical strategies, this conservative choice enabled, however, these institutions to put forward their knowledge on bipolar disorder as reliable and authoritative. This means that the accessibility commitment need not only pose difficulties or bring additional challenges to public institutions. Instead, it might allow such bodies to engage with preferred digital technologies to put forward a desired public image and to bestow their insights in ways that highlight their legitimacy.

Even though both NIMH and HAS used largely similar performative techniques, they approached bipolar disorder in different ways, which seems to confirm yet again that national characteristics and priorities specific to any given healthcare system shape the content public bodies share online. For instance, the higher suicide rate in France (14.3%) as compared to the US (13.1%) (OECD, 2015) may be the reason why HAS chose to perform expertise about bipolar disorder by developing categories of suicide risk and by defining this condition as highly suicidogenic.

Similarly, NIMH's definition of bipolar disorder as a neurological condition is understandable in the American context, where the biomedical model remains dominant and where Congress has been increasingly approving the allocation of funds in areas of research which can provide hard evidence and lead to findings that are easier to render profitable. Nonetheless, while politics play an important role in the functioning and orientation of both agencies, they both successfully managed to relegate it to the backstage, presenting an image of governmental bodies moved by the sole purpose of furthering science and improving the treatment and provision of care to people diagnosed with bipolar disorder.

The analysis discussed here was colored by a specific normative perspective, which sees non-interactive online platforms as rather conservative, whereas interactive online platforms are perceived as more dynamic and amenable to varied purposes. Choosing for an interactive online platform can be problematic for official institutions, because of the inherently generative character of such platforms, where users can engage with the content made available in ways that may lead to interpretations and evaluations of varying quality, and may put forward suggestions that may be detrimental to others. It is regrettable, however, that neither NIMH nor HAS tried to reach a balance between control over the platform and more distributed forms of agency, where users would have had some possibility to contribute, if not to the production, then, at least, to the evaluation of the insights these institutions shared. The need to educate people of different socioeconomic levels and to render insights available to those with disabilities is not a sufficient explanation for their choice of platform type, since online technologies with more open and flexible affordances exist, which can be accessed also from affordable devices. From this point of view, NIMH and HAS' approach is in stark contrast to initiatives developed in recent years in personalized health and e-health (Sardi et al., 2017), where diverse, interactive, gamified elements are integrated to digital technologies and applications to encourage users to engage with the information provided in specific ways. While important reservations exist in regard to such approaches (Lupton, 2020; Prainsack, 2017; Sharon, 2016; Swierstra, 2016; van Dijk et al., 2018) and they need to be carefully considered on a case-by-case basis, the use of interactive online platforms endowed with a diverse array of affordances may help people acquire a better and longer-lasting understanding of complex issues and may further public engagement.

Both NIMH and HAS took up the incentive to share knowledge about bipolar disorder online, but they did so in ways which suggest that they were either oblivious or unwilling to substantially engage with the fact that their authority is questionable and questioned and that they need to convince as experts if they want to succeed in educating their audience. The analysis indicated that whereas HAS had made some efforts toward acknowledging its public accountability, NIMH largely continued to issue pronouncements in a technocratic fashion. While this approach might be a defense mechanism, a way to steer off the public critical climate, it renders these agencies less effective in the convincing provision of insights. Through such practices, they also do not live up to the image they seek to perform online as supporters of public engagement. Whereas this chapter has described how influential governmental agencies performed expertise about bipolar disorder online, in the next chapter I will argue that a particular type of interactive online platform—blogs—allows people diagnosed with bipolar disorder to engage in more substantial ways in processes of knowledge production and evaluation of treatment.

References

Barak, A. (1999). Psychological Applications on the Internet: A Discipline on the Threshold of a New Millennium. *Applied & Preventive Psychology, 8*, 231–245.

Barak, A., & Grohol, J. (2011). Current and Future Trends in Internet-Supported Mental Health Interventions. *Journal of Technology in Human Services, 29*(3), 155–196.

Bennett, G., & Glasgow, R. (2009). The Delivery of Public Health Interventions Via the Internet: Actualizing Their Potential. *Annual Review of Public Health, 30*, 273–292.

Bernstein, R. (2006). A Seat at the Table: Trend or Illusion? *Health Affairs, 25*(3), 730–733.

Bijker, W., Bal, R., & Hendriks, R. (2009). *The Paradox of Scientific Authority. The Role of Scientific Advice in Democracies*. The MIT Press.

Borkman, T. (1997). A Selective Look at Self-Help Groups in the United States. *Health and Social Care in the Community, 5,* 357–364.

Bourdieu, P. (1975). The Specificity of the Scientific Field and the Social Conditions of the Progress of Reason. *Social Science Information, 14*(6), 19–47.

Bureau of Industry and Security (BIS). (2016). *Electronic FOIA.* Accessed August 12, 2017, from https://efoia.bis.doc.gov/

Carlat, D. (2010). *Unhinged: The Trouble with Psychiatry- A Doctor's Revelations About a Profession in Crisis.* Free Press.

Cassani, M. (2017). *Everything Matters. Beyond Meds.* About. Accessed August 12, 2017, from https://beyondmeds.com/about/

Castel, R. (1976). *L'Ordre Psychiatrique. L'Âge d'Or de l'Aliénisme.* Minuit.

Chessick, R. (2006). *The Future of Psychoanalysis.* SUNY Press.

Christensen, H., Griffiths, K., & Jorm, A. (2004). Delivering Interventions for Depression by Using the Internet: Randomized Controlled Trial. *BMJ, 328,* 265–269.

Cyr, D., & Trevor-Smith, H. (2004). Localization of Web Design: An Empirical Comparison of German, Japanese, and United States Web Site Characteristics. *Journal of the American Society for Information, Science and Technology, 55*(13), 1199–1208.

Department of Justice. (2014). Department of Guide to the Freedom of Information Act. *Proactive Disclosures.* Accessed on August 12, 2017.

Desmettre, S. (2009). La Prise en Charge des Troubles Psychiatriques. *Regards Croisés Sur L'Économie, 1*(5), 168–170.

Djonov, E. (2007). Website Hierarchy and the Interaction Between Content Organization, Webpage and Navigation Design: A Systemic Functional Hypermedia Discourse Analysis Perspective. *Information Design Journal, 15*(2), 144–162.

Drucker, J. (2011). Humanities Approaches to Interface Theory. *Culture Machine,* 12. Available at http://www.culturemachine.net/index.php/cm/article/view/434/462

Drucker, J. (2013). Reading Interface. *PMLA, 128*(1), 213–220.

eMEN. (2017). NEWS Summer 2017. Interreg North-West Europe. E-Mental Health Innovation and Transnational Implementation Platform North West Europe: Lille.

Farrell, S., & McKinnon, C. (2003). Technology and Rural Mental Health. *Archives in Psychiatric Nursing, 17,* 20–26.

Felt, U. (2017). Making Knowledge, People, and Societies. In U. Felt, R. Fouché, C. Miller, & L. Smith-Doerr (Eds.), *The Handbook of Science and Technology Studies* (4th ed., pp. 253–257). The MIT Press.

Flemming, J. (1998). *Web Navigation: Designing the User Experience.* O'Reilly Media.

Fussinger, C. (2011). "Therapeutic Community", Psychiatry's Reformers and Antipsychiatrists: Reconsidering Changes in the Field of Psychiatry after World War II. *History of Psychiatry, 22*(2), 146–163.

Gill, K., Kauser, S., Khattack, K., & Hynes, F. (2014). Physician Associate: New Role within Mental Health Teams. *The Journal of Mental Health Training, Education and Practice, 9*(2), 79–88.

Goffman E (1959/1990). *The Presentation of Self in Everyday Life* 8th ed.: Penguin.

Gostin, L. (2008). "Old" and "New" Institutions for Persons with Mental Illness: Treatment, Punishment or Preventive Confinement? *Public Health, 122*(9), 906–913.

Griffiths, F., Lindenmeyer, A., Powell, J., Lowe, P., & Thorogood, M. (2006). Why Are Health Care Interventions Delivered Over the Internet? A Systematic Review of the Published Literature. *Journal of Medical Internet Research, 8*(2), e10. https://doi.org/10.2196/jmir.8.2.e10

Hafermalz, E., Riemer, K., & Boell, S. (2016). Enactment of Performance? A Non-dualist Reading of Goffman. In L. Introna, D. Kavanagh, S. Kelly, W. Orlikowski, & S. Scott (Eds.), *Beyond Interpretivism? New Encounters with Technology and Organization* (pp. 167–181). Springer.

Hilgartner, S. (2000). *Science on Stage: Expert Advice as Public Drama.* Stanford University Press.

Hochmann, J. (2017). *Histoire de la Psychiatrie* (4th ed.). Presses Universitaires de France.

Hopton, J. (2006). The Future of Critical Psychiatry. *Critical Social Policy, 26*(1), 57–73.

Horst, M., Davies, S., & Irwin, A. (2017). Reframing Science Communication. In U. Felt, R. Fouché, C. Miller, & L. Smith-Doerr (Eds.), *The Handbook of Science and Technology Studies* (4th ed., pp. 881–907). The MIT Press.

Horwitz, A., & Wakefield, J. (2007). *The Loss of Sadness. How Psychiatry Transformed Normal Sorrow into Depressive Disorder.* Oxford University Press.

Jongen, H. (2017). *Combating Corruption the Soft Way: The Authority of Peer Reviews in the Global Fight Against Graft.* Datawyse.

Kinderman, P. (2014). *A Prescription for Psychiatry. Why We Need a Whole New Approach to Mental Health and Wellbeing.* Palgrave Macmillan.

Kirsch, I. (2010). *The Emperor's New Drugs: Exploding the Antidepressant Myth.* Basic Books.

Kirsch, I., & Sapirstein, G. (1998). Listening to Prozac but Hearing Placebo: A Meta-Analysis of Antidepressant Medication. *Prevention & Treatment, 1*(2), 0002a. Accessed August 20, 2017, from http://journals.apa.org/prevention/volume1/pre0010002a.html

Knorr Cetina, K. (1999). *Epistemic Cultures. How the Sciences Make Knowledge.* Harvard University Press.

Lane, C. (2009). *Comment la Psychiatrie et L'Industrie Pharmaceutique Ont Médicalisé Nos Émotions.* Flammarion.

Latour, B. (1987). *Science in Action. How to Follow Scientists and Engineers Through Society.* Harvard University Press.

Latour, B., & Woolgar, S. (1979). *Laboratory Life: The Social Construction of Scientific Facts.* Sage.

Levy, J., & Strombeck, R. (2002). Health Benefits and Risks of the Internet. *Journal of Medical Systems, 26*, 495–510.

Loi no. 2005-102 du 11 février 2005 pour l'égalité des droits et des chances, la participation et la citoyenneté des personnes handicapées (1). Accessed August 12, 2017, from https://www.legifrance.gouv.fr/affichTexte.do?cidTexte=JORFTEXT000000809647

Lupton, D. (2020). *Data Selves.* Polity Press.

MacKenzie, D. (1990). *Inventing Accuracy. A Historical Sociology of Nuclear Missile Guidance.* The MIT Press.

Maness, C. (2017). Saving Sigmund: Psychoanalysts Fight to Make Their Profession Relevant. *STAT.* Accessed August 12, 2017, from https://www.statnews.com/2017/03/15/psychoanalyst-freud-relevant/

McLean, A. (2000). From Ex-Patient Alternatives to Consumer Options: Consequences of Consumerism for Psychiatric Consumers and the Ex-Patient Movement. *International Journal of Health Services, 30*(4), 821–847.

McLean, A. (2003). Recovering Consumers and a Broken Mental Health System in the United States: Ongoing Challenges for Consumers/Survivors and the New Freedom Commission on Mental Health. *International Journal of Psychosocial Rehabilitation, 8*, 58–70.

McPherson, S., & Armstrong, D. (2006). Social Determinants of Diagnostic Labels in Depression. *Social Science & Medicine, 62*(1), 50–58.

Metzl, J. (2009). *The Protest Psychosis. How Schizophrenia Became a Black Disease.* Beacon Press.

Ministère Des Affaires Sociales Et De La Santé. (2016, July 4). *Stratégie nationale e-santé 2020.* Paris.

Morrison, L. (2013). *Talking Back to Psychiatry. The Psychiatric Consumer/ Survivor/Ex-Patient Movement*. Routledge.

Moshagen, M., & Thielsch, M. (2010). Facets of Visual Aesthetics. *International Journal of Human-Computer Studies, 68*, 689–709.

O'Sullivan, S. (2016). *It's All in Your Head: True Stories of Imaginary Illness*. Vintage Books.

OECD. (2015). Country Note: How Does Health Spending in FRANCE Compare? *OECD Health Statistics*.

Office of Management and Budget (OMB). (2016). *Memorandum for the Heads of Executive Departments and Agencies*. M-17-06.

Pignarre, P. (2006). *Les Malheurs des Psys. Psychotropes et Médicalisation du Social*. La Découverte.

Potter, J. (1996). *Representing Reality. Discourse, Rhetoric, and Social Construction*. Sage Publications.

Prainsack, B. (2017). *Personalized Medicine. Empowered Patients in the 21st Century?* New York University Press.

Référentiel Général D'Accessibilité Pour Les Administrations (RGAA) Version 3 2017. Accessed August 12, 2017, from https://references.modernisation. gouv.fr/rgaa-accessibilite/

Rissmiller, D., & Rissmiler, D. (2006). Open Forum: Evolution of the Antipsychiatry Movement into Mental Health Consumerism. *Psychiatric Services, 57*(6), 863–866.

Roberts, R., & Itten, T. (2006). Laing and Szasz: Anti-Psychiatry, Capitalism, and Therapy. *Psychoanalytic Review, 93*(5), 781–799.

Romme, M., & Escher, S. (Eds.). (1993). *Accepting Voices*. MIND.

Rose, N. (2018). *Our Psychiatric Futures*. Polity Press.

Sardi, L., Idri, A., & Fernández-Alemán, J. (2017). A Systematic Review of Gamification in E-Health. *Journal of Biomedical Informatics, 71*, 31–48.

Scheid, T. (2000). Rethinking Professional Prerogative: Managed Mental Health Care Providers. *Sociology of Health & Illness, 22*(5), 700–719.

Scott, S. (2006). The Medicalisation of Shyness: From Social Misfits to Social Fitness. *Sociology of Health & Illness, 28*(2), 133–153.

Section 508.gov. *It Accessibility Law and Policies*. Accessed August 12, 2017., from https://section508.gov/manage/laws-and-policies

Shapin S, Schaffer S (1985/2011) *Leviathan and the Air-Pump. Hobbes, Boyle, and the Experimental Life* 2nd ed. : Princeton University Press.

Sharon, T. (2016). The Googlization of Health Research: From Disruptive Innovation to Disruptive Ethics. *Personalized Medicine, 13*(6), 563–574.

Swierstra, T. (2016). Introduction to the Ethics of New and Emerging Science and Technology. In R. Nakatsu, M. Rauterberg, & P. Ciancarini (Eds.), *Handbook of Digital Games and Entertainment Technologies* (pp. 1271–1295). Springer.

Szasz, T. (1961). The Use of Naming and the Origin of the Myth of Mental Illness. *American Psychologist, 16*, 59–65.

The U.S. Digital Service. (2018). *Digital Services Playbook*. Accessed August 12, 2017, from https://playbook.cio.gov/

Van Dijk, J., Poell, T., & de Waal, M. (2018). *The Platform Society*. Oxford University Press.

VPH Institute. (2016). *France National E-Health Strategy 2020*. Accessed August 14, 2017, from http://www.vph-institute.org/news/france-national-e-health-strategy-2020.html

Whitaker, R. (2010). *Anatomy of An Epidemic: Magic Bullets, Psychiatric Drugs, and the Astonishing Rise of Mental Illness*. Crown Publishing Group.

Whitley, R. (2012). The Antipsychiatry Movement: Dead, Diminishing, or Developing? *Psychiatric Services, 63*(10), 1039–1041.

World Wide Web Consortium (W3C). (2017). *Web Content Accessibility Guidelines (WCAG). 2.0*. Accessed August 12, 2017, from https://www.w3.org/TR/WCAG20/

Wright, R., & Cummings, A. (2005). *Destructive Trends in Mental Health. The Well-Intentioned Path to Harm*. Routledge.

Ybarra, M., & Eaton, W. (2005). Internet-Based Mental Health Interventions. *Mental Health Services Research, 7*(2), 75–87.

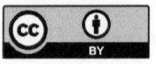

4

Tactical Re-appraisals and Digitally Informed Hypotheses About the Treatment for Bipolar Disorder

While patient engagement in mental healthcare has a long tradition, as already mentioned in the first chapter, since the late 1980s a series of factors has led to a growing responsibilization of people in regard to their health (Petersen & Lupton, 1996) and has stimulated them to contribute to the production of knowledge. The Internet has played an important role in such developments (Wyatt et al., 2013), as it has allowed people diagnosed to enroll in medical studies more easily, to engage in practices of self-monitoring and -experimentation, and to exchange information with more people with the same diagnosis than was previously possible. Yet, while patient engagement is welcomed and encouraged, what exactly is meant by it, what patients are expected to contribute, and what the limits to such contributions are or should be remain debatable (Adams, 2011; Lupton, 2018). These issues are exacerbated online by the variety and specificity characterizing both mental health conditions and online platforms, which shape the content and character of interactions. More

---

The materials used in this chapter from the blog *Bipolar Burble* have been included in an article titled "Bipolar Patients and Creative Online Practices: Sharing Experiences of Controversial Treatments," which was published in the journal *Health*, https://doi.org/10.1177/1363459319838315.

© The Author(s) 2023
C. Egher, *Digital Healthcare and Expertise*, Health, Technology and Society, https://doi.org/10.1007/978-981-16-9178-2_4

research is needed to map out what patients contribute online, and to understand how such contributions are contextually shaped.

Whereas the previous chapter showed how official institutions performed expertise about bipolar disorder, the current one marks the turn in this book toward the various activities undertaken by people diagnosed with bipolar disorder and the different types of expertise they perform online. We remain close to medical perspectives on this condition, however, as this chapter shows how people diagnosed with bipolar disorder use blogs and fora to share their treatment experiences. This way, the role the affordances of online platforms can play in the coordination required for the practical achievement of expertise is highlighted. Using de Certeau's theory (1988) of creative tactics in everyday life, I argue that through their online interactions, they move beyond the performance of lay expertise and collectively generate what I[1] call "digitally informed hypotheses" in areas where the currently available medical knowledge on the effects and side effects of medications is insufficient. In so doing, we will leave behind the focus on how expertise is achieved through the coordination of digital elements on relatively static stages and immerse ourselves in the coordination of exchanges among diverse contributors that are mediated by the affordances of blogs and fora and that underlie the development of these "digitally informed hypotheses."

Problematizing Patient Engagement

People diagnosed with mental health conditions have assumed a growing role in the production of knowledge, as the provision of treatments and caring practices has shifted in the context of deinstitutionalization from medical environments to more private and non-clinical settings, such as homes and community centers. As such, patient engagement in mental healthcare has developed under various forms, ranging from clubhouses and self-help and support groups (McLean, 2003), focusing on the

---

[1] I was inspired to use the term "hypothesis" by some French online contributors, who used this notion to describe a suggestion regarding the effects of certain environmental factors on treatment effectiveness put forward by other people diagnosed with bipolar disorder on the forum *Le Forum des Bipotes*.

societal reintegration of people diagnosed with mental health conditions, to social movements, such as the psychiatric consumer/survivor/ex-patient movement, whose members "attempt to shape treatment to respond to their own needs" (Morrison, 2013: ix). Since the early 1990s, people diagnosed have also participated in the provision of psychiatric care, as paid or voluntary case managers, facilitators, or peer support providers (Davidson, 2005). As such, they have been involved in numerous ways not only in care but also in the production of knowledge about treatment.

More recently, patient engagement has been encouraged through top-down and grassroots initiatives meant to improve the provision of mental healthcare and to render it more cost-efficient. Social media and digital technologies have played an important role in these developments, as they have provided new avenues for patient engagement, which have been both celebrated and critiqued. In the early days of the public Internet, some commentators expected this medium to empower patients, contributing to the re-appreciation of lay expertise (Hardey, 1999). Others have criticized digital technologies as a means for creating free labor, as a neoliberal practice of outsourcing tasks and responsibilities onto individuals while decreasing social provisions (Lupton, 2020; Rose, 2018; Thomas, 2016). Most medical sociologists and media scholars agree, however, that digital technologies have contributed to more active conceptualizations of the role of patients (Felt, 2015). The personal experiences of (pre)patients have become all the more important (Prainsack, 2017), as the adoption of big data analytics in healthcare and the drive toward precision medicine make highly diverse data necessary (Lupton, 2020), including next to traditionally "medical" markers, information such as credit card purchases, and social media interactions (Weber et al., 2014). This has contributed to new perspectives on what counts as evidence (Hogle, 2016) and to intensified calls for individuals to engage in self-monitoring practices and to contribute information.

As the emergence and popularity of movements such as "The Quantified Self" (Lupton, 2016) indicate, many people have responded enthusiastically to such calls and have engaged with numerous digital technologies, such as self-tracking devices, wearables, implantables, and external sensors, to track diverse bodily states, patterns of activities, and moods, thereby contributing to the generation of new types of data.

Most such data have been numerical, thus allowing the users of these technologies to identify patterns in the data, to combine different data sets to arrive at novel insights, and to engage in various comparisons. Depending on their preferences and the available data policies, individuals have thus been able to contribute to the development of new medical knowledge and products in more and less direct ways. Thus, they could share their insights at collective, "show-and-tell" events, such as those organized by supporters of The Quantified Self movement, and they could carefully monitor and provide relevant health data at specific intervals on online platforms such as PatientsLikeMe or CureTogether or participate in various one-person trials (Schork, 2015). But they could also be among the (knowing or unknowing) providers of health data aggregated by initiatives such as IBM Watson Health, the Apple ResearchKit, or Genomera. While researchers and medical professionals have been mainly interested in data generated through digital self-tracking devices, patients and their families have also provided valuable qualitative information, in the form of accounts shared on interactive digital platforms, such as blogs and fora, where they could share their experiences and enrich their knowledge through the narratives provided by other contributors.

Attempts to determine the knowledge of patients have a long history (Segall & Roberts, 1980), and more recently patients' use of online platforms has served to further problematize their relations with medical professionals and to nourish ongoing discussions about the type and relevance of the knowledge each party contributes (Versteeg et al., 2018). While medical knowledge is generally seen as relying upon scientific and clinical insights, patients are often ascribed experiential knowledge, that is, "truth learned from personal experience with a phenomenon rather than truth acquired through discursive reasoning, observations, or reflection on information provided by others" (Borkman, 1976:446).

Two main strands can be distinguished in the debate about the meaning and relevance of patient engagement. Building upon Borkman (1976), one group (Collins & Evans, 2002; 2007; Prior, 2003) focuses on the experiential knowledge of people diagnosed, which they see as stemming from their direct experiences with a condition and argue that such knowledge is different from that acquired formally, through specialized training. Proponents of the other perspective (Arksey, 1994; Epstein, 1995) reject such a strict distinction and highlight the substantial role people diagnosed can play in the development of medical knowledge. Arksey (1994) put forward the notion of "lay expertise" to acknowledge the substantial technical knowledge people could acquire informally. Epstein further developed these insights, showing how some AIDS activists had "learned the language and culture of medical science" (1995:17), and were thereby able to engage in and change medical research and clinical practices. Both positions have shortcomings: while the first perspective conceives of expertise and experience as opposite poles on a continuum, the second runs the risk of expertise being depleted of its substantial character, if applied too generously.

Wilcox (2010) provides a helpful perspective for the analysis in this chapter. She argues that lay expertise should be understood as "collective knowledge that may be widely available yet is still unevenly socially distributed" (2010:45). This is reinforced by studies of health-related online behaviors that have shown that "[s]ocial media platforms facilitate the sharing of health information between users and the co-production of new knowledge that is shaped by personal experience" (Sosnowy, 2014:316). While previously patient associations collected and processed the experiences of numerous individuals diagnosed to transform them into collective knowledge, I argue that such practices are nowadays facilitated by blogs and fora. Authored by one or several individuals and updated regularly, blogs comprise posts on a variety of topics, listed typically in reverse chronological order. Fora are online platforms where individuals can post messages and read those of others along "threads" where insights on a specific topic accumulate, turning fora into rich discussion databases. While on blogs, people diagnosed mainly contribute as reactions to the posts shared by the blog author(s), on fora, even though threads can also be initiated by the forum owner/administrator, they are largely developed by individual users, who want to receive advice on a particular issue. Importantly, both blogs and fora may enable collective processes of knowledge production by bringing together people with the same diagnosis but endowed with different types of knowledge, skills, and resources, by facilitating their dialogue, and by preserving their exchanges. These online platforms are worthy of scholarly attention, since "[h]ealth issues are today often negotiated in parallel with professionals in institutional settings like hospitals and among peers in activities taking place online" (Bellander & Landqvist, 2018:1).

Lay Expertise and Bipolar Disorder

Lay expertise is often articulated in situations when scientific knowledge is lacking, when it has not yet stabilized or when issues are too complex to be solved using only one type of knowledge (Baillergeau & Duyvendak, 2016). This makes its study in relation to bipolar disorder relevant. As already mentioned in Chap. 1, while its causes are not precisely known (Frey et al., 2013), bipolar disorder is thought to be determined by a combination of genetic, neurological, and environmental factors. Treatment is prescribed in a rather formulaic fashion, and there is still limited understanding of how the prescribed medicines work. Finding an effective treatment regimen for any individual patient may take several months or years. In the case of bipolar disorder, therefore, there is a significant amount of space for people diagnosed to contribute to knowledge, making it an interesting site to study patient engagement and the performance of expertise.

According to Britten and Maguire (2016), while medical professionals appreciate patient engagement in various aspects of clinical practice and research, patients' experiences about treatment have not been sufficiently acknowledged. Furthermore, whereas new drugs prescribed for mental health conditions are assessed based on short clinical trials (involving typically six weeks of exposure), many of them are used as maintenance treatment. This means that "the effects of these drugs as used in practice are not known" (Frank et al., 2005: 292) and "decisions about payment, inclusion, placement in formularies and clinical management are usually not informed by data on long-term clinical or economic consequences" (ibid.). What further complicates matters in the field of mental health is that treatment compliance and adherence remain problematic, leading to important tensions between medical professionals and people diagnosed. Nonetheless, in a highly influential study, Martin (2009) has described the complex attitudes people diagnosed with bipolar disorder develop toward their medication and has highlighted the substantial knowledge they have about their own symptoms and reactions to treatment. These are therefore aspects about which people diagnosed with bipolar disorder may be very insightful, and the Internet could provide a welcoming space for those among them who want to share their treatment experiences and contribute to the development of new knowledge.

Studying Tactics Online

Over the last few decades, official institutions have increasingly emphasized the need to inform and consult the public about scientific findings and research agendas. This has contributed to the distribution of scientific information in numerous shapes and across different media. According to Epstein (1996:177), "debates about the safety and efficacy of treatments travel with particular ease between the pages of scientific publications, the mass media…" due to their highly politicized character and the different types of stakeholders involved. Since finding effective treatment is a priority for people diagnosed (Thompson et al., 2012), such debates no doubt reach them, and they may subsequently adapt the information conveyed for their own purposes (Sharon, 2015). The concept of "tactics" developed by de Certeau is therefore useful, as it allows me to analyze the creative ways in which people diagnosed with bipolar disorder take up elements of the dominant discourse regarding the effectiveness of medications, and transform them in their attempts to adjust treatment to their personal needs and preferences. De Certeau (1988: xix) defines tactics as ingenious actions through which individuals seek to re-appropriate dominant representations by adapting them to their own needs, rules, and goals. Tactics "must constantly manipulate events in order to turn them into 'opportunities'" (De Certeau, 1988: xix).

The concept of tactics is pertinent because the online contributions of people diagnosed with bipolar disorder, which I argue that collectively contribute to the development of digitally informed hypotheses, are not always organized and institutionalized, nor do they occur outside the confines of the dominant medical discourse. They rather represent creative practices undertaken from within the dominant order, whereby people diagnosed seek to render the space of medical knowledge about the treatment of bipolar disorder more "habitable." Thus, in the analysis I focus on the perspectives of online contributors, on how current medical views on the treatment of bipolar disorder are understood, taken up, and adapted by them. Tactics are time-bound and therefore appropriate for studying blogs and fora, where people use their creativity and different types of knowledge to interact with others, where the meaning of each individual contribution is co-determined by the content put forward by others, and where it is positioned, in time as well as in space, in relation to it. This concept is also useful because online contributors need to take into account the restrictions imposed on them by platform owners or administrators. Tactics emphasize the malleable, equivocal nature of lay expertise, as the study of blogs and fora makes us more aware of how the engagement with medical insights on bipolar disorder changes depending on the readers' interpretations and needs, and on how the experiences of the contributors putting them forward develop.

Since in de Certeau's framework, tactics represent creative adaptations of dominant representations, I first sought to delineate the main characteristics of current medical knowledge on the treatment of bipolar disorder by engaging with the literature. This involved an initial consultation of relevant sociological studies (Collin, 2015; Healy, 2008; Lakoff, 2005), followed by the review of 30 medical articles published between 2000 and 2016. The characteristics arrived at this way were further refined by reading the abstracts of 15 medical articles published between 2010 and 2018. Three main characteristics were identified and they guided the analysis of the online data.

Online data were gathered from one French and one American interactive platform. *Le Forum des Bipotes* (LFB) is a forum developed by a person diagnosed with bipolar disorder. LFB was founded in 2007 and functioned until 2014. While it is no longer active at the moment, it enjoyed great popularity and it is still maintained online as a source of information. *Bipolar Burble* is the personal blog of Natasha Tracy, who is diagnosed with bipolar disorder. She enjoys celebrity status in this world, as the blogs she has authored have repeatedly been listed among the top best blogs about bipolar disorder, and appear on the first page of results by search engines such as Google. Blogs and fora have the advantage of containing contributions by different stakeholders in relation to bipolar disorder, allowing for a comparison of the ways in which medical information and other types of knowledge are dealt with online by people in different positions of authority and endowed with different resources.

In choosing these online platforms, I aimed to mimic the approach of regular users, and, using the Google index as an indicator of relevance, I limited the selection to the results provided on the first 30 pages. The selection was further refined by excluding multiple pointers to the same item, and by filtering out blogs which were not in English, which had been established for less than one year at the moment when the selection took place (September 2014), and which had few contributors (<10). From these online platforms, I selected 10 entries/threads which covered information on the treatment of bipolar disorder, broadly understood, and which had more than 30 comments each. The data were analyzed using computer-mediated analysis (Herring, 2012) and building upon insights from sociolinguistics (Blommaert, 2005), which highlight the action-oriented and power-laden character of language. An asset in itself, language is also a means to acquire other resources and to achieve specific goals, such as claiming a particular identity, displaying a certain type of expertise, and distinguishing between different claims. For the sake of accuracy, excerpts are reproduced as they appeared online, with no spelling or grammar corrections, and French quotes were translated by the author. As already mentioned in Chap. 1, to respect the privacy of the online contributors and to avoid their identification, their usernames were replaced by pseudonyms and the dates were slightly modified. I will first describe the three characteristics of medical knowledge on the treatment of bipolar disorder identified and will then discuss their re-appropriation on blogs and fora.

Three Characteristics of Medical Knowledge on the Treatment for Bipolar Disorder

Treatment for bipolar disorder focuses on mood stabilization and maintenance and combines medications and psychotherapy. Its prescription occurs in a context where the production and interpretation of clinical evidence remains problematic in mental health, as

[p]sychiatry has a long history of trying to identify predictors of differential pharmacological response, but these attempts began before the evidence-based medicine (EBM) approach was born, were not deployed in the context of RCTs, and were not tested in RCTs. These attempts came from a different tradition, the mechanistic tradition.... (de Leon, 2012: 156)

In the mechanistic tradition, the effectiveness of psychiatric drugs is due to their action upon specific mechanisms in the brain. In the aftermath of the Human Genome Project, the rise of personalized and precision medicine has contributed to numerous attempts to identify genetic markers for bipolar disorder and the biomarkers that render some of the people diagnosed with it responsive to specific treatments. As "the rapid progress in the '-omics' fields makes the notion of evidence a moving target" (Khoury et al., 2008: 1606), nowadays different types of evidence can be produced in multiple, innovative ways, in different settings and involving different stakeholders (Collins & Varmus, 2015). Nevertheless, the studies undertaken thus far have only been mildly successful in providing clear insights on the effectiveness of treatments for bipolar disorder, whereas attempts to identify biomarkers to explain the heterogeneity of drug responses among patients have generally been unsuccessful. Based on the literature review I undertook, I propose that current medical knowledge about the treatment of bipolar disorder is characterized by *uncertainty, complexity, and individualization.*

Uncertainty is "characterized by self-awareness of incomplete knowledge about some aspect of the world" (Han, 2013:16). In the medical field, "[t]he evidence in which different uncertainties are manifest ranges from anecdotal clinical observations to data from randomized clinical trials" (ibid.). Uncertainty about the treatment of bipolar disorder is informed by methodological issues derived from important characteristics of this condition, such as the considerable heterogeneity in the definition and assessment of a mood episode, relapse (Young & Newham, 2006), and therapeutic response. While EBM has led to "an ever-increasing demand for standardization and improved quality in psychiatric treatment" (Geddes & Goodwin, 2001:191), there is still a lot of uncertainty regarding the mechanism of action of various drugs used for the treatment of bipolar disorder. For example, anticonvulsants were introduced in the treatment of bipolar disorder because of certain similarities between this condition and epilepsy, but the current understanding of their action mechanism remains superficial. While the use of any antidepressants in the treatment of bipolar disorder is controversial, studies have reported important variations in their efficacy and tolerability. Yet, there is limited understanding as to the causes of such heterogeneity. Uncertainty also exists in relation to side effects, and this is the case even for substances which have been long prescribed in the treatment of bipolar disorder. For instance, reports on the degree to which long-term lithium use may lead to renal failure or to congenital malformations, when taken during pregnancy, are ambiguous.

Uncertainty is sometimes due to a lack of clarity, but there are also situations when it is due to a gap in knowledge. Various treatment combinations are often prescribed in clinical practice in response to patients' needs, side effects, or other medications they take, while there are no study results available to confirm or discourage such practices. Another type of uncertainty is linked to patient behavior, particularly treatment adherence. For instance, even though lithium is frequently prescribed and is considered to be highly effective for mood stabilization, it may prompt more frequent episodes if it is abruptly interrupted. This is another aspect that renders treatment effectiveness more difficult to define and assess. At the same time, it indicates that treatment decisions need to be based not only on the best available evidence regarding the effectiveness of particular medications, but have to consider treatment adherence and the elements which mostly influence it (Levin et al., 2016).

Complexity denotes the multiple factors which may play a role in the development of a disease and/ or in an organism's reactions to treatment and the awareness that changes in any of these factors may affect others in unpredictable ways, while sometimes remaining themselves hard to foresee (Plsek & Greenhalgh, 2001). In the case of bipolar disorder, complexity is derived from the diverse causes of this condition and the multiplicity of factors involved in its therapeutic approach, which make it difficult to assess the effects of specific elements and interactions and to make informed decisions about treatment. Numerous findings show that the effects of various medications used in the treatment of bipolar disorder not only are influenced by the level of specific hormones and other bodily values but are also importantly shaped by one's genetics (Craddock & Sklar, 2013) and hereditary make-up. For instance, only 30% of people diagnosed with bipolar disorder are responsive to lithium and researchers have been able to develop a general molecular and functional profile of this group. While such responsiveness was thought to indicate a subtype of bipolar disorder, more recent insights suggest that lithium responsiveness is linked with certain symptoms and is heritable (Tighe et al., 2011). Genetic insights indicating that bipolar disorder is not a discrete entity have further contributed to the complexity characterizing the search for treatment, guiding such endeavors across traditional diagnostic boundaries (Harrison et al., 2016). The environment in which one finds oneself provides another complicating dimension (Harrison et al., 2016). Factors such as climate, family situation, workplace stress, and especially shift work, which disrupts night and day rhythms, also influence treatment effectiveness. Comorbidity further complicates current understandings on treatment effectiveness, as medicines prescribed for other conditions may interact with the bipolar disorder treatment, leading either to different effects altogether or to weaker or stronger effects than expected. The timing when particular interventions are used also seems to importantly determine treatment selection and effectiveness. Thus, different medical combinations are considered depending on the condition's developmental stage (Sachs, 2004) and on the age of the people diagnosed. For instance, studies suggest that the use of psychoeducation to prevent relapses is most effective during the first years after diagnosis, with much more modest effects when taken up later (Miziou et al., 2015). Furthermore, the effects of particular medications only become fully manifest after being taken for a long period of time without interruptions.

Individualization understood as individual variations in treatment response has recently come more and more to the attention of researchers (Bates, 2010), and constitutes a move away from "standard" approaches, where reactions to medications are studied among relatively large groups. While the hope is that at some point treatment response will be studied at the level of each person of interest, individualization currently denotes practices which focus on subgroups of increasingly smaller sizes, as distinctions are made at greater levels of specificity. From this perspective, attempts at determining treatment effectiveness in the field of mental health have also been strongly influenced by developments in the field of pharmacogenetics, as various studies have shown that determining a patient's genotype can help when deciding upon the prescription of specific antipsychotic drugs (Tanaka & Hisawa, 1999). At the same time, various studies have focused on how and why particular subgroups diagnosed with bipolar disorder react differently to specific substances, requiring higher or lower dosages for the intended effects. Insights from personalized medicine have led to a growing awareness that evidence about treatment effectiveness requires taking into account parameters such as dosage, form, and frequency and that genetic, hereditary, and environmental factors may trigger different reactions in different individuals (Hedgecoe & Martin, 2003). Developments in genetics have prompted medical researchers to hope that genetic loci playing a role in the development of bipolar disorder will be found, leading to the identification of biomarkers and to the development of more effective treatment pathways and targets (Squassina & Pisanu, 2013). There has also been a growing recognition that "an individual's unique life circumstances… influence disease susceptibility, phenotype, and response to treatment" (Ziegelstein, 2015: 888). Next to genetic or genomic markers, various personal categories, many of which are dynamic and change numerous times throughout the life of a particular individual (Naylor & Chen, 2010), have thus come to play a role in the development of knowledge about the treatment of bipolar disorder. This way, the evidence about treatment effectiveness has been expanded to include "psychological, social, cultural, behavioral, and economic factors of each person" (Ziegelstein, 2015:888).

In the remainder of this chapter, I will show that such realizations are not restricted to the pages of academic publications, but reach people diagnosed with bipolar disorder, who engage with them both to achieve practical goals and to contribute to the development of new knowledge.

Engaging with Medical Knowledge About the Treatment of Bipolar Disorder Online

The analysis of the online data revealed that people diagnosed were aware of current medical knowledge on the treatment of bipolar disorder, as the following three tactics were identified: the mobilization of the notions of uncertainty, complexity, and individualization. Rather than being merely neutral spaces where these exchanges unfolded, I argue that blogs and fora allowed for individual hunches or suppositions to thicken into what I call "digitally informed" hypotheses about new factors that may influence the effectiveness of treatment. As we will see below, the narrative format specific to contributions on such platforms enabled people diagnosed with bipolar disorder to describe in great detail their various states, to select the aspects each of them found important and meaningful to share in the absence of pre-set rubrics and criteria, and to convey contextual information and aspects of the qualities of their experiences that generally resist quantification. This way, online contributors could provide more clues about the applicability and relevance of their insights, they engaged dialogically in the assessment of the views and experiences shared by others, and they used different, additional standards to evaluate the credibility of various statements.

The design and affordances of blogs and fora played an important role in the development of "digitally informed hypotheses." Thus, they enabled online contributors to engage in various interactive practices whereby personal views or assumptions could solidify and acquire a more general character: by liking specific contributions, by directly reacting to them through comments and expressing similarities of experience, and by providing hyperlinks to studies and other resources in their support. Furthermore, blogs and fora allowed for the longitudinal accumulation in the same space of similar experiences, even when conveyed through fleeting exchanges by occasional contributors. This made possible the gradual emergence of a limited body of evidence, pointing to fruitful areas for further inquiry or, as was mostly the case here, self-experimentation. Whether or not certain personal insights turned into collectively generated hypotheses was often a question of repetition, accumulation, and visibility. This process was thus not only informed by the urgency of the aspects under discussion, but also informed by how skillfully various online contributors could mobilize online affordances and by the flexibility allowed by the platform owners/administrators. The latter were influential through the various rules they set regarding the type of content that could be made available, the word limit for each contribution, and the modality in which insights could be shared. Worth to be mentioned here are, for instance, Tracy's decisions to provide links on her blog's homepage to the blog entries with the highest number of comments and to those with the most recent comments, which kept them in the attention of her audience and increased the likelihood that they would accumulate more contributions. The curatorial work the forum administrator engaged in also shaped the visibility of some insights, as he moved comments made on the one thread onto another which he considered more suitable, and re-positioned certain threads on the first page of the forum when major social and cultural events suggested they would be of interest. Thus, "digitally informed hypotheses" about the effects and side effects of medications emerged as online contributors re-appropriated the notions of uncertainty, complexity, and individualization through interactions mediated by the technologies of blogs and fora.

Uncertainty

People diagnosed sought to address medical uncertainty about the effects of certain substances by engaging in self-experiments. In so doing, they mobilized uncertainty through their ability to locate and manipulate important gaps in relevant medical knowledge, both at the scientific and clinical level, thereby identifying a space which could mainly be furbished through the insights they provided. For instance, in a post from October 2011, Tracy argued that a certain chemical substance might be a new cheap and effective supplement in the treatment of bipolar depression. She cautioned, however, that, while promising, the evidence was limited. In the aftermath, her readers tried this substance, kept careful track of their reactions to it, and shared their experiences at different moments in time:

I started taking it about 6 months ago after reading your blog about it. I have had no side effects and have had no depressive episodes either. I have had a mixed episode but the depressive symptoms were much less than they would normally be. I'm still cautious about saying it has helped and still monitoring but so far so good. Thank you for mentioning it in the first place. We are all different and some people may have negative effects, that's the same with anything. I would say give it a go. (Jane, November 7, 2014)

*

I've been taking [substance name] for about 18 months now, I have had no side effects, the depressions have not been as bad and I think possibly the highs are less too. I do get psychosis and I haven't noticed any effect on this. Although my doctor is sceptical I will continue to take it. Hopefully if the trials are successful doctors will be more likely to suggest this treatment. This same doctor recommended glucosamine for my arthritis so it's not that he is against supplements. (Jane, November 19, 2015)

Something akin to a hierarchy or an attempt at a systematic assessment becomes apparent in both comments, as *Jane* focuses first on the presence or absence of side effects, then on this substance's effects on depression, for which it is intended, and only later on its impact on other symptoms. While the first quote testifies to the influence online bloggers have upon their readers' treatment, both excerpts suggest that people diagnosed make sense of their experiences with medications in a relational way. In her first contribution, *Jane* solves the dissonance between her findings and those of other people diagnosed by invoking the uniqueness of each person and echoes Tracy in recommending it to others. In her second comment, experiential and medical knowledge are described as being at odds with each other, as *Jane*'s tentatively positive findings and intention to continue taking the pills are set against her doctor's doubts. Given *Jane*'s awareness about the limited amount of clinical evidence available, her sharing activity and encouragement for others to try this substance may be seen as an attempt to help fill these gaps in medical knowledge. The mild improvements she describes further suggest that she may make treatment decisions using lower effectiveness standards than medical professionals. Medical uncertainty may therefore be a cause for hope in certain instances and may help to keep people diagnosed motivated and actively engaged with their treatment.

French online contributors re-conceptualized uncertainty to test medical claims about the benefits some of the medications they took for bipolar disorder could have upon other bodily processes. Thus, various online contributors shared insights which they had acquired from their doctors about the neuroprotective effects of lithium, as well as their own opinions and experiences in this respect:

> This is what my shrink says:
> Lithium protects against Alzheimer's. For my mother this seems to be true thus far....
> (....)
> Sometimes I don't know who or what to believe... (Oliane, September 7, 2012)

At the time when contributions such as this were made, the mechanisms through which lithium achieved its neuroprotective effects remained unclear (Forlenza et al., 2014). The available evidence about these effects was largely derived from preclinical trials and from retrospective registry studies conducted on people diagnosed with bipolar disorder. Whereas *Oliane* invoked the psychiatrist as well as the experiences of her mother to legitimate the claim about lithium's neuroprotective effects, it gradually acquired more credibility, as more contributors confirmed having heard about these effects, and having taken the claim seriously enough to base treatment decisions on them:

> I've also heard this about Alzheimer's, and also for multiple sclerosis. (Kat, September 8, 2012)
> *
> My psychiatrist at the expert center in Marseille says that lithium reconstitutes the neural connections that explode under the effect of bipolarity. It also protects from Alzheimer's disease.
> These arguments have tipped the scales even for me, who am a rebel when it comes to taking drugs. I agreed to resume a lithium treatment. I'm starting tonight. He also prescribed Xéroquel. But to that one I say no! I'm still fighting it. (Annemarie, September 8, 2012)

The highest level of credibility ascribed to this view was provided by *Bipote_Admin*, who referred to lithium's neuroprotective properties as a fact:

> Apart from that, as Annemarie says, the neuroprotective and even trophic effect of lithium is worth mentioning because it opens up new therapeutic perspectives. An increase in the volume of gray matter, especially in the frontal lobe, has been observed in patients undergoing lithologic therapy. A thymic episode is neurotoxic and its repetition can cause neurobiological damage. (Bipote_Admin, September 8, 2012)

The use of medical terminology and the passive voice serve to render this claim more credible and neutral. The last sentence echoes the views NIMH put forward that we discussed in the previous chapter, and it indicates that Bipote_Admin's insights were informed by an understanding of bipolar disorder as a brain condition. Since many of the clinical studies which had confirmed this hypothesis were based on neuroimaging techniques (Bearden et al., 2007; Machado-Vieira et al., 2009), this can be seen as an indication of the degree to which this online contributor had internalized medical knowledge.

The excerpts above show that reframing uncertainty in terms of tactics is helpful to understand how people diagnosed with bipolar disorder negotiate medical knowledge to turn their personal experiences into valuable contributions. Other complex factors that can influence treatment effectiveness are discussed below.

Complexity

People diagnosed with bipolar disorder mobilized the notion of complexity online, as they sought to put forward new factors informing variations in the effectiveness of medications. Not content with merely describing the particular effects they experienced, online contributors actively sought confirmation or additional information from others regarding these experiences, often so that they could use such insights as resources to better negotiate with medical professionals in favor or against the prescription of specific medications. Generics were often mentioned in such contexts by American online contributors. For instance, they invoked the complexity of interactions between the various substances contained in this type of medicines and the role variation in their different dosages may have to put forward the hypothesis that their effectiveness varied:

> Ugh! This weekend I picked up a refill (…) At home, I realized the pills looked different. I took them but experienced NO relief whatsoever. I took the bottle down to the pharmacy and insisted they were not what I had been receiving only to be told they WERE. I know what I take and what my pills look like after all this time. A second visit with another pharmacist at the same pharm told me that indeed they had switched generics on me. Did you know that the FDA allows a 20–30% variable amount of the active ingredient in generics. I did not until LOTS of research. You have to be your own doctor AND pharmacist, apparently… (Marina, October 6, 2014)

Marina's comment depicts this hypothesis as the outcome of a discovery journey and traces this contributor's development from the classical "good patient" described by Freidson (1970), who was willing to comply with medical advice even when the pills looked differently, to more recent understandings of patienthood, which conceive of people diagnosed as interested in educating themselves about their condition and assuming an active role in its management. The unfolding of the events described in this quote further serves to reinforce the unbiased character of *Marina's* claims, as she only became distrustful when confronted with an embodied experience—the pills' lack of effect—and set out to find out more information about generics, their compositions, and pharmaceutical regulations once this experience was legitimated by a "traditional" expert. That people diagnosed with bipolar disorder take up the role of investigators to make sense of their personal experiences about medication is illustrated by one of the reactions to *Marina's* contribution:

> My doc told me it's a 40 percent swing… Issue is the filler… Different manufacturers use different fillers which can effect how the med is used by your system. Some can come on strong while others are weak… Many braded pills have 10 manufacturers or more and they are mostly overseas. The FDA could give a hoot. I find that most pharmacists know very little also… Probably because they have so many different meds

to deal with… And, if you notice many generics have gone up in price tremendously since the branded aren't available…Money. Money, Money. (Jack, October 6, 2014)

This exchange illustrates how people diagnosed take up a potential factor an online contributor suggested to influence the effectiveness of medication and try to make sense of it building upon their own experiences and insights. In this case, the varying effectiveness of generics is confirmed and further explanation for it is sought not only by considering the different action of the chemical compounds used, but also by relating it to their manufacturers and to the more or less strict legislation existing in the countries where they are based. Importantly, these comments indicate that online contributors ascribe the limited or incorrect information they receive from different sources to different causes: some unintentional and due to systemic issues, such as the pharmacists having a hard time to keep up with all the new types of medications available, while others intentional and due to corruption, such as official bodies failing to intervene due to their close ties with the pharmaceutical industry. Since the latter are depicted as mainly motivated by commercial interests, the hypotheses people diagnosed develop based on their personal experiences about treatment acquire more credibility among online contributors. The failure of certain governmental agencies to involve and inform the public in more effective ways about their regulatory procedures may thus have a negative impact on their public image and contribute to shifts in the tasks and cognitive authority of different stakeholders. In this context, people diagnosed with bipolar disorder may become more influential and succeed in re-positioning themselves in relation to medical professionals and even researchers through their more active engagement in the production of new knowledge and through the existence of an audience willing to take their insights into account.

People diagnosed with bipolar disorder also re-appropriated the notion of complexity to refine medical insights about some of the factors influencing treatment effectiveness. This was, for instance, the case for a, certain atypical antipsychotic which is recommended to be taken with a meal. Whereas in her blog post Tracy described recent study results which specified the number of calories required per meal for this medicine to be effective, online contributors further specified these insights by arguing that not only the number of calories influenced treatment effectiveness, but also the types of proteins consumed, as the following quote illustrates:

> I don't know the correct spelling [of medication] (…) I have this med down to a science. I eat a homemade hamburger … at 12:30 p.m. and then I drink a small chug of milk at 1:15 p.m. and then finally another hamburger and glass of skim milk at 1:45 p.m. If you eat the second hamburger and glass of milk any earlier than 1:45 p.m. it will not work and you will be sick for the next 12 hours. Then you must repeat the process at 12:30 a.m. You also cannot drink any water after taking [name of medicine] until you wake up. You can take one swig of water here or there but I try not to. One thing that has worked for me is not eating or drinking anything from 9:30 until 12:30. [name of medicine] is a trial and error drug and I have schooled my doctor on what works. (Watson, March 9, 2015, quote slightly adapted to ensure anonymity)

Striking here is the level of detail and precision provided by *Watson*, whose claim to expertise is based on the substantial knowledge he acquired through the varied tinkering practices that he engaged in to fine-tune what he considers to be the most effective approach to the intake of this medicine. Even though *Watson* spells the name of this medication wrongly, his recommendation is bracketed at the beginning and at the end by his claim to scientific authority, which is further emphasized by the description of a reversal in positions between himself and his doctor. Such statements serve to increase the legitimacy of the insights *Watson* provides, whereas the dissonance between his incorrect spelling and the authoritative character of his statement suggests that he may consider practical knowledge, with which he believes to be endowed, more important than abstract, theoretical insights.

Other online contributors re-appropriated the complexity of symptoms of bipolar disorder to advocate for an expansion of therapeutic interventions, so as to include, next to various combinations of medical treatments and "talk" therapies, elements of interior design, atmospheric aspects, such as air pressure and humidity, and the use of specific objects:

> Have you done EMDR [Eye Movement Desensitization and Reprocessing]? What about a Sun Lamp? There is 1 on Amazon by Sphere Technologies

that is $69. It has the highest reviews on Amazon. My friend lent me one and I have been using it for a 8 days. You want to get one that is 10,000 lux and I have seen them as low as $49. (…) I think the sun lamp is worth a shot. It's primarily made for people with SAD [seasonal affective disorder]. I am also going to start volunteering at the animal shelter as a "Cat Socializer". You just go and play with the cats and it makes you feel better, and of course the cats too, and makes them more adoptable. (*Roger,* April 11, 2015)

This quote suggests that for this particular contributor personal experiences as well as the evaluations provided by others on online platforms such as Amazon constitute reliable evidence in favor of taking up potentially therapeutic procedures. At the same time, *Roger* is dedicated to providing other contributors with accurate insights, as he carefully situates his claims by mentioning for how long he had been using the sun lamp and by clearly stating that it was primarily developed for another condition. The details about the price of this technology and how he came to use it are illustrative of the financial considerations that people diagnosed with bipolar disorder who live in the US need to take into account when evaluating their treatment options, and were echoed by many other contributors.

The comparison between the French forum and the American blog revealed that these considerations were importantly shaped by social and cultural factors. While the effectiveness of generics or the cost of objects ascribed therapeutic value were important topics among online contributors in the US, they were not mentioned by French contributors, whose insurance coverage spared them such worries. Furthermore, the analysis of the online data suggested that the blog studied here was at times an important venue through which American contributors, who were no longer insured, could benefit from up-to-date insights on available treatments, as they gained access to medical information. Online exchanges thus came to replace, to a certain extent, medical encounters, as some uninsured online contributors, who had to pay out of pocket for medication, used the treatment experiences and information shared by others to determine what medication would be most effective for them. In contrast, American and French contributors who were insured claimed to have other motivations for engaging in online exchanges. Thus, some wanted to share the insights they acquired on the factors affecting the effectiveness of treatment with their doctors, whereas others wanted to determine whether or not to contact other medical professionals when their own doctors were away or, in some cases, to figure out whether their experiences were serious enough to warrant disturbing their doctor while on holiday.

The tactics through which American and French online contributors re-appropriated complexity were also influenced by national institutional perspectives on mental health. It was thus obvious that many online contributors on the French forum supported a biopsychosocial model of disease, which, as I mentioned in the previous chapter, was the dominant approach to mental healthcare in France up until the early 2000s, as they emphasized the need to tackle bipolar disorder by addressing it simultaneously as a biological, psychological, and social condition. In general, French contributors advocated an understanding of treatment effectiveness as not solely the result of the actions of the various chemical substances they took, but also of the various types of therapies and social support available. Furthermore, many of the additional therapies they suggested had a dialogical or interactional character, such as psychoanalytic approaches and eye movement desensitization and reprocessing therapy. While "talk" therapy or Alcoholics Anonymous (AA) meetings were often mentioned by American contributors, approaches focusing on dietary changes and on technological interventions, such as vagus nerve stimulation (VNS) and even electroconvulsive therapy (ECT), were by far more popular. At the same time, a pronounced overreliance on medications could be noted, which some of the blog contributors were aware and critical of:

> You miss 1 day of your Seroquel, or your Cymbalta, or your Depakote… seriously, it will be okay… if not, use your psychotherapy techniques. Oh, that's right… not too many actually do psychotherapy… it's all the meds baby. (*Mandy*, May 12, 2011)

Overall, both American and French online contributors argued in favor of acknowledging a more diverse array of chemical interactions and practices as influencing treatment effectiveness. Personal preferences also informed the choice of therapeutic intervention, and they are discussed below.

Individualization

People diagnosed with bipolar disorder creatively engaged with medical insights about individualization in treatment response to argue for the recognition of diverse personal preferences and leisurely pursuits as important influences on treatment effectiveness. For researchers, such variations refer to the identification of specific, small(er) groups sharing common molecular, environmental, and personal attributes. In contrast, online contributors often interpreted individualization so that each person's health and illness trajectory became unique, which sometimes prompted them to argue against evidence derived from RCTs. In such instances, they advised others not to focus too much on statistics, but to bear in mind that the challenges they were facing were deeply personal and unlike those of anyone else.

In general, online contributors re-interpreted individualization to argue that lifestyle choices or leisurely activities which fell outside of the medical domain had therapeutic value, and often engaged in comparisons between their effects and those of medications, as the quote below illustrates:

> Recently (I did something very random though less so for my brain), as I was coming out of a big depression, I went horse-riding, a great passion … well this session was the equivalent of an antidepressant and an anxiolytic, I was in the seventh heaven … Zen, feeling well … and this word 'well', we often look for it in our illness.
>
> The therapeutic effect: it stimulates, it "zenifies", it has an anti-depressant effect without a change of mood!
>
> You and other bipolars shook me up, my shrink as well … but very frankly I didn't want to listen… I had to find the "drive", to set the machine in motion again…
>
> For the moment I have found it again… and I am much better. (*Sunset*, Xeroquel, August 7, 2011)

This contributor seems to suggest that the pursuit of a hobby might be better than the categories of medications invoked, since its anti-depressive effects are not accompanied by the risk of mania or hypomania. The suggestion that leisurely pursuits have therapeutic effects is strengthened in the second part of the quote, where the state of well-being thus acquired is reported to be lasting. Other people diagnosed with bipolar disorder took up this suggestion and contributed to its development into a hypothesis, by reporting similar positive effects they were experiencing when engaging in their favorite activities, be they reading, cooking, or contributing on online platforms:

> this blog and your collective experiences have been better for me than any medications as they usually have side-effects that are not welcomed. (*Damian,* February 25, 2014)

While these comments may indicate that the borders between the treatment and (self)management of a condition are rather porous for the people diagnosed with bipolar disorder studied here, only some of these digitally informed hypotheses have thus far coincided with scholarly interest. The last two quotes refer to practices that have been more successful from this point of view. For instance, whereas a focus on horses has been missing thus far in therapeutic approaches to bipolar disorder, this topic has received more attention over the last few years in relation to autism (Malcolm et al., 2018). Similarly, the idea that participation in online support communities would have positive effects on the well-being of a person diagnosed is the object of ongoing research. Whereas some of the results produced thus far have been inconclusive (Lagan et al., 2020; Naslund et al., 2016), others give some cause for hope that digital interactions with certified peer specialists can improve treatment outcomes in mental healthcare (Fortuna et al., 2019).

Unlike the contributors discussed above, another group of people diagnosed with bipolar disorder also re-interpreted individualization in treatment response by using the degree to which they could engage in activities that were meaningful to them as new and, arguably, more relevant standards to assess treatment effectiveness. In such instances, they went beyond considerations as to whether or not a certain medication stabilized their mood, and focused, instead, on the extent to which it allowed them to perform social roles, professional duties, or activities they enjoyed, be that the joy of interacting with their children, to fulfill their athletic aspirations, or to have a body image more aligned to their personal aesthetic ideals. Such accounts succeeded in rendering the effects of specific treatments "thick," meaningful, understandable to people diagnosed as well as undiagnosed. In so doing, they helped others decide whether a certain medicine or therapeutic approach might be worth a try, based on similarities in life circumstances, hobbies, personal values, and preferences.

The identification of successful treatments according to such individualized standards was often accompanied by effusive displays of gratitude and appreciation:

> I bless every day the medical team who discovered the effects of lithium, even though I'm suffering from its toxicity to the kidneys today, and I don't regret having taken this treatment over a long period of time. I owe it the best years of life, calmer and more serene than I could have imagined. (*honeysuckle*, September 19, 2012)

As this quote indicates, such enthusiasm was not only reserved for medications with minimal side effects or where the side effects had not yet become apparent, but emerged as the result of a careful retrospective analysis. The accumulation of superlatives attached to the positively qualifying adjectives in the second sentence is illustrative of the ways in which affective markers functioned as indicators of the degree of confidence online contributors had in the effectiveness of medications. Unlike scientific accounts of treatment assessment which steer away from sentimentality and subjectivity, people diagnosed with bipolar disorder used sentimental effusions judiciously, but they did mobilize them for specific medications, to lend additional persuasive strength to their accounts about treatment effectiveness. Given that individual perceptions were accepted as reliable and authoritative by the other contributors, this reframing of individualization might contribute to heighten the epistemic relevance of emotional and affective personal markers in a field where authoritative knowledge has traditionally been acquired based on groups and the calculation of averages.

Other online contributors re-appropriated individualization to suggest that personality traits, one's attitude toward treatment, and the level of personal commitment could impact on the effectiveness of medical treatment. Thus, in numerous comments the role of personal characteristics, such as risk aversion, tolerance, patience, and curiosity, on treatment response was seriously considered. This is, for instance, how a contributor made sense of the absence of positive effects the first time she took lithium:

> I think the first time I wasn't patient enough. I was expecting too much, too quickly. I don't really know what it means to be balanced and I was expecting an influx of positive emotions. Until then I had only seen life in black, in gray ... so I wanted to see it in pink, at least from time to time. Whereas normal life is not like that at all! And it's true that I'm used to being constantly overwhelmed by emotions. I thrive on adrenaline. I think I have never known anything else, because the disease appeared too early. I don't even know what it's like to live normally ... to live without having to struggle, without making any excesses. That's why I didn't think that I was that sick! By force of habit! (*Annemarie,* September 8, 2012)

This excerpt suggests that the performative effect of expectations (Engel & Van Lente, 2014) is also applicable when it comes to embodied experiences, as in *Annemarie's view,* individuals need to be ready for certain medications and experienced enough to recognize when they are effective. Making the right decisions about treatment is thus not only understood as a matter of one's mental and physical state, but also depends on the time of onset of the disease and the degree of self-knowledge that one had by then acquired, a point to which we will return in Chap. 5. *Annemarie* further points to an important element which informs treatment non-adherence among people diagnosed with bipolar disorder, as some of them enjoy their (hypo)manic states and have a hard time appreciating (clinical) stability, which they experience as a flattening of affect. It thus illustrates that lay expertise is not only a matter of acquiring vast experiential knowledge combined with medical insights, but that it also entails the capacity to manage one's expectations, to acquire a better understanding of what living with bipolar disorder when receiving effective treatment can feel and look like.

Overall, online contributors mobilized individualization to provide insights meant to enable other people diagnosed with bipolar disorder to decide upon treatment, depending on their lifestyle preferences, on what they appreciated most about their existence and wanted to maintain, restore, or improve. They thus rendered the space of medical knowledge about treatment meaningful to them by inscribing in it elements and experience they found fulfilling. The implications of these findings are discussed below.

Discussion

People diagnosed with mental health conditions have been actively engaged in their health for a long time. In a context where medical knowledge has permeated different areas of society, and has, thus, become amenable to multiple usages and interpretations, the Internet provides new avenues for them to exchange insights and to contribute to the production of knowledge. Using de Certeau's (1988) theory of creative tactics it has been possible to show that people diagnosed with bipolar disorder develop more nuanced positions than challenging or accepting medical perspectives online, to take their insights and suggestions about treatment effectiveness seriously, and to approach them as productive exchanges which may lead to new knowledge. Thus, by mobilizing the notions of uncertainty, complexity, and individualization, online contributors sought to state the importance of individual experiences as epistemic resources, to put forward new factors influencing treatment effectiveness, and to advocate for an expansion of therapeutic interventions. In so doing, I have argued that they went beyond the performance of lay expertise and collectively developed "digitally informed hypotheses" about treatment effectiveness in an attempt to render the space of their interactions with medical professionals and of daily life with bipolar disorder more comfortable. The findings discussed in this chapter thus contribute to a substantial body of literature which has highlighted the value of blogs in providing people diagnosed with more tailored resources to navigate daily life (Adams, 2010) and the Internet's ability to facilitate collective learning and the development of epistemic communities (Akrich, 2010).

The epistemic practices described here took place in a context marked by a broadening of the conceptualization of health-relevant data, as the growing number of wearable technologies people use and the digital traces they leave behind has made available tremendous amounts of information. Yet, unlike individuals who engage with digital self-tracking tools as "interpreters of the body" (Lupton, 2013), online contributors on the blog and forum studied relied upon other people diagnosed with bipolar disorder as their sounding board, as they made sense of the various states, moods, and other insights they collected dialogically. As we will discuss in more detail in Chap. 5, these activities support an understanding of such interactive online platforms as spaces for biosociality (Kingod, 2018), where contributors share their experiences and the creative practices they develop to better manage their conditions (Pols, 2014). The design and affordances of blogs and fora importantly shaped the development of "digitally informed hypotheses," as the coordination required for such epistemic practices was facilitated through the repetition, accumulation, and visibility of particular ideas over extended periods of time that they allowed for. The fact that information from different years can be located in the same place has, however, potential drawbacks, as proximity on the blog or forum might obliterate important contextual factors, and unreflectively equate experiences shaped by specific temporal and social coordinates. This may have negative consequences for the reliability of the inferences made based on such insights, as they may lack internal consistency, but also on their validity, since elements that are important to correctly interpret the data used are missing or not taken into consideration. While the de-contextualized use of data is already common in data analytics, many scholars have warned against the consequences such practices may have upon the quality of the scientific claims inferred from them and about the societal transformations they may lead to (Gregory et al., 2019; Prainsack, 2017; Wyatt et al., 2013).

Through their comments, contributors showed that the effects of medications do not manifest themselves in pristine laboratory conditions but occur in the messy context of daily life of people with the same diagnosis, but perhaps with different symptoms, bodily reactions, needs, and preferences. They also suggested that the effects and side effects of medications are shaped by the specific circumstances of the lives they act upon, and such knowledge is still insufficient at the medical level. While the recommendations of medical professionals are based on evidence obtained in conditions where high levels of validity and reliability can be guaranteed, the online interactions between people diagnosed with bipolar disorder indicate that they often value insights acquired through the accumulation of personal accounts, whose reliability is indicated through detailed descriptions and the presence of affective and emotional markers next to medical information. These perspectives are in line with findings which suggest that medical professionals and people diagnosed have contrasting views on knowledge and validity (Bellander & Landqvist, 2018), and which argue that "[t]he epistemic authority of the patient's experience as a source of knowledge emerges not in spite, but precisely because, of its highly emotive and embodied dimensions" (Mazanderani, 2014:141).

The comparison of the tactics through which American and French online contributors re-appropriated medical uncertainty, complexity, and individualization as treatment response revealed important similarities and differences. Both French and American online contributors engaged in online exchanges to achieve specific pragmatic goals, as they tried to identify more suitable treatments for themselves depending on their lifestyle and personal preferences, to expand the meaning of treatment to include various practices, or to consider its effects in interaction with a more complex array of substances and activities. They also tried to acquire more agency in their interactions with medical professionals by having their experiences confirmed by many others. The analysis further indicated that cultural, social, and institutional differences importantly shape online contributions, leading to noteworthy distinctions. More cross-cultural studies on the treatment experiences of people diagnosed with bipolar would be highly valuable, as they would cast light upon important similarities and differences in reactions hitherto considered as mainly biological, and may reveal what factors inform them.

While this chapter discussed how people diagnosed with bipolar disorder contributed collectively to the development of new insights about treatment effectiveness, the next one will show that the ideal of active patienthood combined with the skillful use of the Internet and an entrepreneurial spirit can render some individuals diagnosed with bipolar disorder highly influential. One of these individuals is Natasha Tracy, who in this chapter received limited attention as the owner of the blog from which data were collected, but who will come into the limelight due to another position she occupies and a more substantial engagement in expertise about bipolar disorder.

References

Adams, S. (2010). Blog-based Applications and Health Information: Two Case Studies That Illustrate Important Questions for Consumer Health Informatics (CHI) Research. *International Journal of Medical Informatics, 79*, 89–96.

Adams, S. (2011). Sourcing the Crowd for Health Services Improvement: The Reflexive Patient and "Share-Your-Experience" Websites. *Social Science & Medicine, 72*(7), 1069–1076.

Akrich, M. (2010). From Communities of Practice to Epistemic Communities: Health Mobilizations on the Internet. *Sociological Research Online, 15*(2), 10. Available at http://www.socresonline.org.uk/15/2/10.html

Arksey, H. (1994). Expert and Lay Participation in the Construction of Medical Knowledge. *Sociology of Health & Illness, 16*(4), 448–468.

Baillergeau, E., & Duyvendak, J. W. (2016). Experiential Knowledge as a Resource for Coping with Uncertainty: Evidence and Examples from the Netherlands. *Health, Risk & Society, 18*(7–8), 407–426.

Bates, S. (2010). Progress Towards Personalized Medicine. *Drug Discovery Today, 15*(3), 115–120.

Bearden, C., Thompson, P., Dalwani, M., Hayashi, K., Lee, A., Nicoletti, M., & ...Soares, J. (2007). Greater Cortical Gray Matter Density in Lithium-Treated Patients with Bipolar Disorder. *Biological Psychiatry, 62*(1), 7–16.

Bellander, T., & Landqvist, M. (2018). Becoming the Expert Constructing Health Knowledge in Epistemic Communities Online. *Information, Communication & Society, 23*(4), 507–522. https://doi.org/10.108 0/1369118X.2018.1518474

Blommaert, J. (2005). *Discourse: A Critical Introduction.* Cambridge University Press.

Borkman, T. (1976). Experiential Knowledge: A New Concept for the Analysis of Self-Help Groups. *Social Service Review, 50*(3), 445–456.

Britten, N., & Maguire, K. (2016). Lay Knowledge, Social Movements and The Use of Medicines: Personal Reflections. *Health, 20*(2), 77–93.

Collin, J. (2015). Universal Cures for Idiosyncratic Illnesses: A Genealogy of Therapeutic Reasoning in the Mental Health Field. *Health, 19*(3), 245–262.

Collins, H., & Evans, R. (2002). The Third Wave of Science Studies. Studies of Expertise and Experience. *Social Studies of Science, 32*(2), 235–296.

Collins, H., & Evans, R. (2007). *Re-thinking Expertise*. Chicago: The University of Chicago Press.

Collins, F., & Varmus, H. (2015). A New Initiative on Precision Medicine. *New England Journal of Medicine, 372*(9), 793–795.

Craddock, N., & Sklar, P. (2013). Genetics of Bipolar Disorder. *The Lancet, 381*, 1654–1662.

Davidson, L. (2005). Recovery, Self Management and the Expert Patient-Changing the Culture of Mental Health from a UK Perspective. *Journal of Mental Health, 14*(1), 25–35.

de Certeau, M. (1988). *The Practice of Everyday Life*. University of California Press.

De Leon, J. (2012). Evidence-based Medicine Versus Personalized Medicine: Are They Enemies? *Journal of Clinical Psychopharmacology, 32*, 153–164.

Engel, N., & Van Lente, H. (2014). Organizing Innovation and Control Practices: The Case of Public-Private Mix in Tuberculosis Control in India. *Sociology of Health and Illness, 36*(6), 917–931.

Epstein, S. (1995). The Construction of Lay Expertise: AIDS Activism and the Forging of Credibility in the Reform of Clinical Trials. *Science, Technology & Human Values, 20*(4), 408–437.

Epstein, S. (1996). *Impure Science: AIDS, Activism, and the Politics of Knowledge*. University of California Press.

Felt, U. (2015). Sociotechnical Imaginaries of "the Internet", Digital Health Information and the Making of Citizen-Patients. In S. Hilgartner, C. Miller, & R. Hagendijk (Eds.), *Science and Democracy: Making Knowledge and Making Power in the Biosciences and Beyond* (pp. 176–197). Routledge.

Forlenza, O., De-Paula, V., & Diniz, B. (2014). Neuroprotective Effects of Lithium: Implications for the Treatment of Alzheimer's Disease and Related Neurodegenerative Disorders. *ACS Chemical Neuroscience, 5*(6), 443–450.

Fortuna, K., Brook, J., Umucu, E., Walker, R., & Chow, P. (2019). Peer Support: A Human Factor to Enhance Engagement in Digital Health Behavior Change Interventions. *Journal of Technology in Behavioral Science, 4*, 152–161.

Frank, R., Conti, R., & Goldman, H. (2005). Mental Health Policy and Psychotropic Drugs. *The Millbank Quarterly, 83*(2), 271–298.

Freidson, E. (1970). *The Profession of Medicine.* Harper and Row.

Frey, B., Andreazza, A., Houenou, J., Jamain, S., Goldstein, B., Frye, M., et al. (2013). Biomarkers in Bipolar Disorder: A Positional Paper from the International Society for Bipolar Disorders Biomarkers Task Force. *Australian & New Zealand Journal of Psychiatry, 47*(4), 321–332.

Geddes, J., & Goodwin, G. (2001). Bipolar Disorder: Clinical Uncertainty, Evidence-Based Medicine and Large-Scale Randomised Trials. *The British Journal of Psychiatry, 178*(S41), 191–194.

Gregory, K., Cousijn, H., Groth, P., Scharnhorst, A., & Wyatt, S. (2019). Understanding Data Search as a Socio-Technical Practice. *Journal of Information Science, 46,* 1–17. https://doi.org/10.1177/0165551519837182

Han, P. (2013). Conceptual, Methodological, and Ethical Problems in Communicating Uncertainty in Clinical Evidence. *Medical Care Research and Review, 70*(1), 14–36.

Hardey, M. (1999). Doctor in the House: The Internet as A Source of Lay Health Knowledge and the Challenge to Expertise. *Sociology of Healthy & Illness, 21,* 820–835.

Harrison, P., Cipriani, A., Harmer, C., Nobre, A., Saunders, K., Goodwin, G., & Geddes, J. (2016). Innovative Approaches to Bipolar Disorder and Its Treatment. *Annals of the New York Academy of Sciences, 1366*(1), 76–89.

Healy, D. (2008). *Mania: A Short History of Bipolar Disorder.* John Hopkins University Press.

Hedgecoe, A., & Martin, P. (2003). The Drugs Don't Work. *Social Studies of Science, 36,* 723–752.

Herring, S. (2012). Discourse in Web 2.0.: Familiar, Reconfigured, and Emergent. In D. Tannen & A. Tester (Eds.), *Georgetown University Round Table on Languages and Linguistics 2011: Discourse 2.0.: Language and new media* (pp. 1–29). Georgetown University Press.

Hogle, L. (2016). Data-intensive Resourcing in Healthcare. *BioSocieties, 11*(3), 372–393.

Khoury, M., Berg, A., Coates, R., Evans, J., Teutsch, S., & Bradley, L. (2008). The Evidence Dilemma in Genomic Medicine. *Health Affairs, 27*(6), 1600–1611.

Kingod, N. (2018). The Tinkering M-Patient: Co-Constructing Knowledge on How to Live with Type I Diabetes Through Facebook Searching and Sharing and Offline Tinkering with Self-Care. *Health,* 1–17.

Lagan, S., Ramakrishnan, A., Lamont, E., Ramakrishnan, A., Frye, M., & Torous, J. (2020). Digital Health Developments and Drawbacks: A Review and Analysis of Top-Returned Apps for Bipolar Disorder. *International Journal of Bipolar Disorders, 8*(39), 1–8.

Lakoff, A. (2005). *Pharmaceutical Reason. Knowledge and Value in Global Psychiatry.* Cambridge University Press.

Levin, J., Krivenko, A., Howland, M., Schlachet, R., & Sajatovic, M. (2016). Medical Adherence in Patients with Bipolar Disorder: A Comprehensive Review. *CNS Drugs, 30*(9), 819–835.

Lupton, D. (2013). Quantifying the Body: Monitoring and Measuring Health in the Age of mHealth Technologies. *Critical Public Health, 23*(4), 393–403.

Lupton, D. (2016). *The Quantified Self. A Sociology of Self-Tracking.* Polity Press.

Lupton, D. (2018). *Digital Health.* Routledge.

Lupton, D. (2020). *Data Selves.* Polity Press.

Machado-Vieira, R., Manji, H., & Zarate, C. (2009). The Role of Lithium in the Treatment of Bipolar Disorder: Convergent Evidence for Neurotrophic Effects as a Unifying Hypothesis. *Bipolar Disorder Suppl., 2*, 92–109.

Malcolm, R., Ecks, S., & Pickersgill, M. (2018). 'It just opens up their world': Autism, Empathy, and the Therapeutic Effects of Equine Interactions. *Anthropology & Medicine, 25*(2), 220–234.

Martin, E. (2009). *Bipolar Expeditions. Mania and Depression in American Culture* (2nd ed.). Princeton University Press.

Mazanderani, F. (2014). The Patient's View: Perspectives from Neurology and the 'New' Genetics. *Science as Culture, 23*(1), 135–144.

McLean, A. (2003). Recovering Consumers and a Broken Mental Health System in the United States: Ongoing Challenges for Consumers/Survivors and the New Freedom Commission on Mental Health. *International Journal of Psychosocial Rehabilitation, 8*, 58–70.

Miziou, S., Tsitsipa, E., Moysidou, S., et al. (2015). Psychosocial Treatment and Interventions for Bipolar Disorder: A Systematic Review. *Annals of General Psychiatry, 14*(19), 1–11.

Morrison, L. (2013). *Talking Back to Psychiatry. The Psychiatric Consumer/Survivor/Ex-Patient Movement.* Routledge.

Naslund, J., Aschbrenner, K., Marsch, L., & Bartels, S. (2016). The Future of Mental Health Care: Peer-To-Peer Support and Social Media. *Epidemiology and Psychiatric Sciences, 25*(2), 113–122.

Naylor, S., & Chen, J. (2010). Unraveling Human Complexity and Disease with Systems Biology and Personalized Medicine. *Personalized Medicine, 7*(3), 275–289.

Petersen, A., & Lupton, D. (1996). *The New Public Health. Health and Self in the Age of Risk.* Sage.

Plsek, E., & Greenhalgh, T. (2001). Complexity Science: The Challenge of Complexity in Health Care. *BMJ, 323,* 625–628.

Pols, J. (2014). Knowing Patients: Turning Patient Knowledge into Science. *Science, Technology & Human Values, 39*(1), 73–97.

Prainsack, B. (2017). The "We" in the "Me": Solidarity and Health Care in the Era of Personalized Medicine. *Science, Technology, & Human Values, 43*(1), 21–44.

Prior, L. (2003). Belief, Knowledge and Expertise: The Emergence of the Lay Expert in Medical Sociology. *Sociology of Health & Illness, 25,* 41–57.

Rose, N. (2018). *Our Psychiatric Futures.* Polity Press.

Sachs, G. (2004). Strategies for Improving Treatment of Bipolar Disorder: Integration of Measurement and Management. *Acta Psychiatrica Scandinavica, 110*(S422), 7–17.

Schork, N. (2015). Personalized Medicine: Time for One-Person Trials. *Nature, 520,* 609–611.

Segall, A., & Roberts, L. (1980). A Comparative Analysis of Physician Estimates and Levels of Medical Knowledge Among Patients. *Sociology of Health & Illness, 2*(3), 317–334.

Sharon, T. (2015). Healthy Citizenship Beyond Autonomy and Discipline: Tactical Engagements with Genetic Testing. *BioSocieties, 10*(3), 295–316.

Sosnowy, C. (2014). Practicing Patienthood Online: Social Media, Chronic Illness, and Lay Expertise. *Societies, 4,* 316–329.

Squassina, A., & Pisanu, C. (2013). Personalized Medicine in Bipolar Disorder: How Can We Overcome the Barriers to Clinical Translation? *Personalized Medicine, 10*(8), 765–768.

Tanaka, E., & Hisawa, S. (1999). Clinically Significant Pharmacokinetic Drug Interactions with Psychoactive Drugs: Antidepressants and Antipsychotics and the Cytochrome P450 System. *Journal of Pharmacy and Therapeutics, 24*(1), 7–16.

Thomas, P. (2016). Psycho Politics, Neoliberal Governmentality and Austerity. *Self & Society, 44*(4), 382–393.

Thompson, J., Bissell, C., Cooper, C., Armitage, C., & Barber, R. (2012). Credibility and the "Professionalized" Lay Expert: Reflections on the Dilemmas and Opportunities of Public Involvement in Health Research. *Health, 16*(6), 602–618.

Tighe, S., Mahon, P., & Potash, J. (2011). Predictors of Lithium Response in Bipolar Disorder. *Therapeutic Advances in Chronic Disease, 2*, 209–226.

Versteeg, W., Te Molder, H., & Sneijder, P. (2018). "Listen to Your Body": Participants' Alternative to Science in Online Health Discussions. *Health, 22*(5), 432–450.

Weber, G., Mandl, K., & Kohane, I. (2014). Finding the Missing Link for Big Biomedical Data. *JAMA, 311*(24), 2479–2480.

Wilcox, S. (2010). Lay Knowledge: The Missing Middle of the Expertise Debates. In R. Harris, N. Wathen, & S. Wyatt (Eds.), *Configuring Health Consumers. Health Work and the Imperative of Personal Responsibility* (pp. 45–64). Palgrave Macmillan.

Wyatt, S., Harris, A., Adams, S., & Kelly, S. (2013). Illness Online: Self-Reported Data and Questions of Trust in Medical and Social Research. *Theory, Culture & Society, 30*(4), 131–150.

Young, A., & Newham, J. (2006). Lithium in Maintenance Therapy for Bipolar disorder. *Journal of Psychopharmacology, 20*(2), 17–22.

Ziegelstein, R. (2015). Personomics. *The Journal of the American Medical Association Internal Medicine, 175*(6), 888–889.

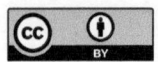

5

Online Expert Mediators: Expanding Interactional Expertise

Blogs are interesting. They show that humans want to communicate. They show that we want to share our stories. They also became money making opportunities and vanity projects that sometimes make me question my own motives. I am VERY careful about what I share. I am personal without over-sharing. I'm careful of my brand. I protect it every day. I know what I write and I know the effect it has on my audience. (Fast, May 8, 2017, e-mail interview)

This is how Julie A. Fast, one of the best-known bloggers on bipolar disorder and a person who, based on her own admission, has helped shape this genre, describes this type of interactive online platform and her engagement with it. This quote is impressive in its honesty and it also highlights specific opportunities the Internet has contributed to as well as the need for a particular type of expertise to be able to take advantage of them. This chapter is dedicated to the study of interactional expertise,

---

A modified version of this chapter will be published in the special issue "Expertise and Its Tensions" in *Science and Technology Studies*. Whereas the chapter focuses on two bloggers—Natasha Tracy and Julie A. Fast—in the article, the online and offline activities of another blogger—Charlotte Walker—are also discussed.

© The Author(s) 2023
C. Egher, *Digital Healthcare and Expertise*, Health, Technology and Society,
https://doi.org/10.1007/978-981-16-9178-2_5

focusing on the activities of two highly successful bloggers diagnosed with bipolar disorder. Whereas in the previous chapter one of them figured in her function of platform owner, shaping the conditions of possibility for other people diagnosed with bipolar disorder to contribute online, here their personal substantial engagement in the development of new knowledge will be focused on. In so doing, the relevance of the multiple and shifting positions that stakeholders can occupy in relation to the development of expertise, which is foregrounded in the new conceptualization thereof that I put forward, will be highlighted.

Relations between important stakeholders in the field of mental health have been significantly transformed by the Internet (Barak & Grohol, 2011). This medium has affected the identity and the type of interactions between knowledge producers and users (Wyatt et al., 2013), contributing to the diversification of sources of medical knowledge away from clinical environments (Nettleton, 2004), closer to the everyday settings of people diagnosed (Lucivero & Prainsack, 2015), and leading to the re-appreciation of other types of knowledge (Schaffer et al., 2008). Such changes have taken place in a context where pronounced neoliberal tendencies have introduced a market logic in the provision of healthcare and have encouraged individuals to assume responsibility for their health (Novas, 2006; Rose, 2007). Web 2.0 technologies enable users not only to consume information but also to engage in its production (Lupton, 2014). Thus, the current dominant imperatives to stay or become healthy by seeking and sharing health-related information have contributed to the development of a space where new forms of agency can develop (Kivits, 2013). Whereas the previous chapter has shown how people can perform lay expertise and collectively contribute new insights about bipolar disorder, the focus shifts here to the new entrepreneurial subjectivities (Tutton & Prainsack, 2011) that these technologies have contributed to. By studying the activities of two bloggers using Collins and Evans' (2002) concept of interactional expertise, I show that through their skillful use of the Internet, some individual patients have become highly influential, and argue that this medium has thus helped facilitate the emergence of a new type of stakeholder—the online expert mediator. In so doing, I expand the notion of interactional expertise by arguing that it has more of a bi-directional nature than Collins and Evans (2002) and

Collins et al. (2017) assume and that it is important to consider the effects of the medium through which it is performed. But first, let us consider how the role of patients in mental health has changed over the last few decades, focusing on the Internet's influence in these transformations.

Greater Mental Health Patient Engagement and the Internet

As many medical sociologists have indicated, since the last few decades of the twentieth century patient engagement has been promoted in different areas and for different goals (Barello et al., 2014; Turner, 1995), through top-down processes (Godfrey et al., 2003; Hogg, 2009) or as a result of grassroots activities (Barbot & Dodier, 2002; Kushner, 2004; Landzelius, 2006; Novas, 2006; Rabeharisoa et al., 2013; Taussig et al., 2003). The meaning and consequences of patient engagement vary (Hickey & Kipping, 1998; Rowland et al., 2017), yet, as the findings in the previous chapter show, people diagnosed have also come to grasp the conditions of complexity and uncertainty under which medical professionals operate, leading to a growing awareness of the limits of medical expertise. These realizations have had a profound resonance in mental health, where the authority of medical professionals has been challenged since the late 1960s (Pickersgill, 2012), in manners which were discussed in more detail in the introductory chapter. Combined with official restructuring initiatives and considerable openness among people diagnosed toward new approaches and types of knowledge, such challenges have contributed to the proliferation and diversification of mental health professionals (Brown, 1988; Grob, 2005). The relations between existing stakeholders have thus been modified, and the role of patients has changed from passive recipients of care (Barnes & Shardlow, 1997) to consumers who feel entitled to choose the type of care they receive (McLean, 2000). While some patients consider themselves survivors and actively militate against medical conceptualizations and interventions (Crossley & Crossley, 2001; Speed, 2006; Whitley, 2012), many others have engaged in processes of knowledge production (Gillard et al., 2012; Kemp, 2010), evaluation (Director, 2005), and implementation (Davidson, 2005), thereby acquiring a greater role in mental health.

People diagnosed have used the Internet for different types of epistemic engagements. Some patients have used the knowledge thus acquired to question and/or challenge the expertise of medical professionals in several ways (Fox et al., 2005; Gowen et al., 2012; Mulveen & Hepworth, 2006; Orsini & Smith, 2010). Others have engaged in various scientific activities, ranging from monitoring themselves using self-tracking devices and sharing their data with others to using collaborative platforms, such as PatientsLikeMe, to test medical hypotheses (Kallinikos & Tempini, 2014). Through their use of the Internet, such "citizen scientists" or "health hackers" have gone beyond the mere provision and exchange of medically interesting information, connecting with other people with the same diagnosis to "conduct clinical trials on their own diseases" (Bottles, 2013:88), thereby enacting particular values and ideals of patienthood (Sharon, 2017). Such online opportunities have been all the more important in the field of mental health, where study participation has traditionally been difficult, as the symptoms of people diagnosed often rendered their adherence to specific interventions problematic, while the desire to avoid stigmatization made them reluctant to attend face-to-face meetings (Naslund et al., 2015).

Used in mental health since its early days, the Internet has importantly shaped the participation of people diagnosed in knowledge production. Already in 1999, Barak (1999: 231) noted that "the rapid developments in computers and information technology over the past decade have had an impact on psychology, which has moved (...) from local computer applications to network applications that take advantage of the Internet." By now, numerous studies have indicated the potential (Barak et al., 2008; Carlbring & Andersson, 2006; Proudfoot, 2004; Smith et al., 2011) and variety of online interventions for mental health (Barak & Grohol, 2011; Kraus et al., 2010; Marks et al., 2007; Ybarra & Eaton, 2005). Bipolar disorder is among the mental health conditions affected by such approaches, as various online therapies and different types of mobile phone applications have been developed (Nicholas et al., 2015).

There are important differences in approach, motivation, and goals among patient organizations focusing on the same condition (Barbot, 2006) and even among members of the same group (Epstein, 1996). The Internet has helped render more visible the heterogeneity of bipolar patients, as various online platforms testify to their different needs and preferences. It has also contributed to the emergence of new types of involvement for people diagnosed with bipolar disorder, by diversifying the range of stances at their disposal. By using the Internet, they have been able to develop new skills and to acquire various resources. This has not only rendered bipolar patients more salient stakeholders, but it has also contributed to a diversification of the type of stakeholdership they could take up.

Since the emergence of surveillance medicine in the twentieth century (Armstrong, 1995), and particularly after the adoption of a consumerist culture in healthcare (Lupton, 1995), individuals have been encouraged to engage in self-surveillance practices and to actively manage their health by staying informed. The development of digital technologies has contributed to the diversification and intensification of these tendencies (Kopelson, 2009), but has also "promoted the individual expression of a personal experience of health" (Kivits, 2013:222), as people have been increasingly exhorted not only to seek information but also to share personal insights. Thus, the Internet has enabled not only patient groups, but also individuals to become influential by achieving high levels of visibility and by acquiring numerous readers. While most researchers have studied the changing identity and growing influence of patients as a result of collective actions, several academic works have highlighted the importance of particular individuals in shaping the character of patient organizations and of their interactions with medical professionals (Klawiter, 1999; Lerner, 2001). This chapter makes a contribution in this sense, by showing that some individual patients have become highly influential in mental health by taking advantage of some of the opportunities generated by the development of Web 2.0 platforms in the context of growing tendencies to responsibilize individuals for their health (Nettleton, 2004).

Among the multiple forms of self-expression the Internet has enabled, illness blogs represent a highly popular genre (De Boer & Slatman, 2014). Given their popularity, malleable architecture, and primarily individual character, blogs represent an excellent site to study the activities, knowledge practices, and alliances through which individuals achieve an influential position. Illness blogs are a specific type, as they "are used to express the experience of illness and to connect with readers via the internet" (Heilferty, 2009:1542). They differ based on their design, accessibility, and interactive character, and it is the more or less skillful combination of affordances related to these aspects that largely determines a blog's standing.

Two Bloggers on Bipolar Disorder

On December 3, 2016, an online search using the keywords "bipolar blog" generated 12,600,000 results on Google and 6,870,000 on Yahoo. Regardless of the search engine used, the blog of Natasha Tracy, which was discussed from a different perspective in the previous chapter, and of Julie A. Fast came up on the first page of results, either directly or mentioned under rubrics such as "the best bipolar blogs of the year" on several health platforms. They are thus likely to come to the attention of many Internet users, especially since both of them can be accessed freely by readers.

Each of these bloggers has been diagnosed with bipolar disorder for about two decades. Tracy is an award-winning mental health speaker and writer on topics such as bipolar disorder, depression, pharmacology, and other mental health–related issues. She has authored three blogs—*Breaking Bipolar*, *Bipolar Burble*, and *Bipolar Bites*—and has been a contributor to the *Huffington Post*. Her blogs attract large numbers of visitors, and many of her posts receive hundreds of comments. Fast is "a world leading mental health expert on the topics of bipolar disorder, depression, seasonal affective disorder, personality disorders and mood management." She states that her site and blog together have been visited by one million visitors. Unlike Tracy, her personal blog, *Bipolar Happens!*, only gathers a very modest number of comments (< 10), but there is significantly more interaction on her blog on the bipolar disorder "Hope" magazine website, *Fast Talk*. Fast also works as a "bipolar disorder management specialist" at Share.com, the website created by Oprah and Dr. Oz. To reach audiences of different ages, in recent years, Fast has also actively engaged in the provision of information about bipolar disorder on Instagram and Facebook.

While Internet users have been studied as health-related information seekers and/or producers, less attention has been paid to their potential as information mediators. Illness blogs are important mediation sites, as experiential knowledge is combined with medical, pharmaceutic, and socioeconomic information. These bloggers function as mediators, as they "transform, translate, distort, and modify" (Latour, 2005:39) the information they share in order to adapt it to the opportunities and limitations of the medium and to the requirements of different audiences (Wathen et al., 2008). Importantly, the development of this new stakeholder category occurs in a context where patient experiences have come to be valued, elicited in various ways online, and, subsequently, commodified (Adams, 2013; Lupton, 2014; Mazanderani et al., 2012). I argue that through their practices and collaborations with different stakeholders, these two bloggers move beyond the role bipolar patients generally have in the field of mental health, and turn themselves into a new type of stakeholder—the online expert mediator.

Theoretical Approaches to Interactional Expertise

The online activities of these bloggers are analyzed instead using the concept of interactional expertise (Collins & Evans, 2002), which bridges the divide between practical, experiential, and scientific knowledge. This notion is particularly useful, because it allows me to identify people endowed with substantial knowledge but missing official credentials, and provides an appropriate explanatory framework when studying phenomena "involving different expert communities" (Collins et al., 2017: 782). While contributory expertise denotes one's ability to contribute productively to a field (Collins & Evans, 2007), interactional expertise "is expertise in the *language* of a specialism in the absence of expertise in its *practice*" (emphasis in the original) (Collins & Evans, 2007: Loc. 520).

This means that people endowed with interactional expertise have specialist tacit knowledge and they understand the language of a domain of practice and can engage in interesting conversations with those with contributory expertise in that domain, but they cannot make practical contributions to it. Thus, people may acquire interactional expertise through immersion in a field while following a different trajectory than contributory experts (Collins et al., 2006). Interactional expertise is also highly specific: just like contributory experts in a field can contribute successfully only in some areas, interactional experts can be more competent about particular subdomains of a field. Furthermore, the acquisition of interactional expertise enables people to function as mediators between contributory experts in a field and the group(s) they represent.

Collins and Evans (2015, 2017) have studied interactional expertise using the Imitation Game, which is an adaptation of the test Alan Turing developed to assess the intelligence of computers. In so doing, they resist calls to expand the initial definition of interactional expertise in ways which they believe would diminish its "real" character. Nevertheless, in this chapter I follow the lead of scholars who have argued for a broadening of the way in which this concept is understood (Goddiksen, 2014). I thus take up Plaisance and Kennedy's (2014) recommendation to study interactional expertise by considering the "fruitful" contributions people endowed with it can bring to a field due to "the various profiles that interactional experts can have as a result of who they are, why they've sought to acquire IE [interactional expertise], and how they make use of it" (Plaisance & Kennedy, 2014:65). In so doing, I extend interactional expertise by considering the effects of taking seriously the medium through which it is displayed and I show that it has more of a bi-directional character than Collins and Evans had envisaged.

I argue that there are important differences between the activities people can engage in and the approaches that they can choose from to display interactional expertise, depending on the medium they use. While some people may be able to understand their interlocutors better and express themselves more eloquently during face-to-face encounters, they may have a more difficult time displaying their interactional expertise convincingly via the telephone, in writing, or online. Furthermore, each medium might bring them in touch with different audiences, with different criteria for assessing credibility, different expectations, and informational needs. By studying the activities of Tracy and Fast on different online platforms, I identify various ways in which these bloggers make use of online affordances in order to successfully deploy interactional expertise and thereby establish themselves as authoritative figures in the field.

These two bloggers were identified using the Google index as a relevance indicator, as I aimed to mimic the approach of regular users. Data were collected between July 2014 and September 2018 and initially consisted of bloggers' posts about the treatment of bipolar disorder and information provided under the "about" rubric of every blog. To acquire a better understanding of the bloggers' standing and other public activities, additional online queries were subsequently conducted, using the bloggers' names as search terms in the search engine Google. The search "Natasha Tracy" generated 19,600,000 results, while "Julie A. Fast" 349 million. The biographical and social data were collected from the first ten pages of results. I also conducted an e-mail interview with Julie A. Fast and an online interview with Natasha Tracy using the Skype telecommunications application. I performed thematic analysis of all the texts collected, including hyperlinks and images, by identifying important themes through repeated readings (Lupton, 1995). I operationalized interactional expertise based on Collins and colleagues' approach (2006) into three main dimensions: linguistic fluency in the field of medical knowledge about bipolar disorder; ability to evaluate and distinguish between medical professionals; and ability to provide practical advice about relevant matters in the field. Given the aim of expanding the notion of interactional expertise, the following aspects were additionally focused on how and when bloggers invoked and displayed medical knowledge; the bloggers' relations with medical professionals; the alliances they forged; elements conveying the bloggers' standing; and the bloggers' use of online affordances. In what follows, I discuss how these bloggers have turned themselves into online expert mediators.

Tracing the Development of a New Stakeholder Category

Technical Prowess

A first characteristic of online expert mediators is their endowment with or access to substantial technological skills. Fast and Tracy managed to become online expert mediators because they were among the first to realize the Internet's potential and to understand how much people diagnosed with bipolar disorder needed their insights. While Tracy has a degree in computer science and used to work for Microsoft, Fast's long-term partner at the time when she started sharing her perspectives on bipolar disorder online was a gifted programmer. She also mentioned that both of them were technology enthusiasts. In the e-mail interview I conducted with her, Fast stated that her "internet career was a perfect storm of events" (Fast, May 8, 2017, e-mail interview) and noted the role that various technologies and her partner's abilities to make use of them played in her career:

> In that EXACT moment in the spring of 2002, I had the idea that I could take my first two books and sell them as download books. No one was doing this except a few guys who were selling sales tools and real estate guides. I found NO books on the internet about any psychology topic or even any self help topics. I knew I had a good idea. (…) We spent the next month building a website to sell my two books. I turned my manuscripts into PDF files and because he was a programmer and a computer genius-we were able to build something that hardly existed at the time. An ebook website! The books were Bipolar Happens! and my Health Cards Treatment System for Bipolar Disorder. I wrote a home page- Ivan created links for people to buy the books through something called a SHOPPING CART and the business was born. It wasn't that long ago, but can you believe that the words Ebooks and shopping cart were so new, we were not even sure what they meant. My business helped define the process. I <u>was the first person in the world to sell a psychology or self help ebook online.</u> (my emphasis)

I say it was a perfect storm because on the exact month that I started my webpage, Google started something new called ADWORDS. I was one of their first customers. I created an ADWORDS account and started to advertise my treatment plan from the first week it was online. This was perfect timing. Believe me, so much of what happens online is LUCK. Yes, I was prepared and I had a truly great product, but the timing was perfect. Often, you have to be in the right place in order to adapt new technology. (Fast, May 8, 2017, e-mail interview)

In this blogger's view, therefore, her considerable influence is partly due to her innovative approach and the active role she played in the development of the field of self-help e-books from its inception.

Both bloggers credit their success to the specific character of online communication and digital technologies, which allowed them for advance planning and for the content they created to be made available to their audiences regardless of their health state at any given moment in time. Fast mentioned, "I was sick a lot- so having an internet business was a miracle for me. I could be sick and still sell my books" (Fast, May 8, 2017, personal communication), and argued that "[a]n internet business is the ONLY business I can do considering my brain limitations" (Fast, May 8, 2017, e-mail interview). At the same time, the bloggers emphasized that different online platforms afford varying degrees of control and power and that appropriate skills have to be acquired to use each type of platform to one's benefit:

THEN, Facebook happened. I can't tell you enough how this changed everything. MySpace simply couldn't do what Facebook did. Facebook made talking about yourself very easy. I had a love/hate relationship with Facebook for many years. I was bullied a lot and didn't know how to control the flow of information. Webpages and blogs are safe spaces- the author controls who says what. Facebook was a free for all. It was amazing and destructive at the same time. I now know exactly how to use it, but it's an art. I can say the same for Twitter. (Fast, May 8, 2017, e-mail interview)

To render their online undertakings successful, the bloggers also had to call upon different types of knowledge and make wise decisions about the involvement of other professionals. Just as the Internet is multiple, so are the skills necessary to use it in one's favor, and developing such insights requires time and numerous other resources that few people may have at their disposal. Reflecting on the important role of website statistics in her online activities, Fast stated:

> It's important to know that the internet is incredibly ALIVE- we do things that you can't do in a regular business…So many internet business owners make decisions that are creative instead of business oriented *and* creative. You need both. Creative people who don't really like looking at stats tend to just post and hope for the best. In reality, a successful internet entrepreneur always has the business in mind and must look at stats from every source possible. It's an ever changing environment, but stats are always the friend of an online business. You can hire someone to do this, but you need to understand it yourself first. (Fast, March 20, 2021, personal communication)

Next to statistics, timing and the early development of relevant relationships seem to have been of great importance for the online careers of these bloggers. Fast's early start using one particular online technology enabled her to be among the first to embrace many others, which allowed her to increase her online visibility: *"I also feel… these three sites [her sales website, her PR page, and her blog] have helped with Google rankings"* (Fast, May 23, 2017, personal communication). From this other point of view, these online technologies also contributed to important inequalities, as her status as a successful early adaptor provided her with more authority and influence than people who started using them later, thereby enabling her, based on her own admissions, also to shape the genre of illness blogs.

Interactional Expertise

Next to technical skills, Fast and Tracy also needed to develop and perform interactional expertise about medical knowledge on bipolar disorder to successfully function as online expert mediators. The display of linguistic fluency in a field is the main mark of people endowed with interactional expertise (Collins & Evans, 2002). While Tracy and Fast are not medical professionals, nor did they study medicine, the many years since they have been diagnosed with bipolar disorder, the multitude of treatments they have tried, and the great variety of professionals they have consulted have provided them with ample opportunities to observe the practices of the medical community. Furthermore, their own proactive attitudes have enabled them to deepen their medical knowledge about bipolar disorder. These bloggers display their linguistic prowess throughout their posts and interactions with commentators, as they explain medical phenomena using a more accessible vocabulary and providing examples, they give advice about the most appropriate therapeutic approaches depending on one's symptoms and/or life circumstances, and they are aware of the latest developments in the field. The excerpt below is illustrative of such activities:

> Drug tolerance is also known to occur upon drug-discontinuation. In other words, someone who has previously responded well to lithium discontinues the drug, symptoms reemerge, the person goes back on lithium but does not find it effective. Again, we don't know why this occurs but it does appear to in a small percentage of patients. In one study, it occurred in 13.6 percent of people taking lithium.
>
> (…)
>
> Warning, this is a preclinical study and as such the implications from it may not be fully understood. Please make sure to make any medication changes only with doctor oversight. For more information please see the study Tolerance to the Prophylactic Effects of Carbamazepine and Related Mood Stabilizers in the Treatment of Bipolar Disorders [hyperlink provided]. (Tracy, Bipolar Bites, May 30, 2012)

This quote indicates Tracy's position as mediator between medical professionals and bipolar patients, a position which I argue is characteristic for this new type of stakeholder. While it may be that it refers to the level of knowledge available to the whole of humanity, the use of "we" in a context where study results are discussed suggests that Tracy sees herself more as a member of the medical community. At the end of the post, however, she reclaims her subordinate position to medical professionals, while by sharing the source she used, Tracy reveals her awareness of the need to legitimize her claims.

Mediators importantly transform the meaning of the information they transmit, and this is obvious in the posts authored by both bloggers. While they convincingly use medical vocabulary, they do so in particular ways. For instance, in a manner which reiterates the tactic of individual-ization discussed in the previous chapter, Tracy puts forward her own reading of personalized medicine, as on numerous occasions she seems to believe that each person displays an individual mix of symptoms and reacts differently to treatment, as the quote below illustrates:

> And if 99 people say the med is bad, but 1 says it's good, what benefit is that? Should the patient not try it? Should the patient assume the med won't work or will have too many side effects? The 99:1 ratio essentially means nothing because we're all different. (Tracy, Breaking Bipolar, June 30, 2011)

Furthermore, Tracy often uses statistics and results obtained through randomized controlled trials to support her claims. This shows that she makes strategic choices about the ways in which she refers to medical information, an approach previously identified among patient organiza-tions (Treichler, 1999). This rather complicated balancing act is necessary as it allows her not to alienate readers with experiences different from the ones she describes while maintaining her authority. At the same time, it enables her not to stray too far from the prevailing medical consensus, thereby retaining her ties with the medical community.

The bloggers display their linguistic prowess also by distinguishing between different medical professionals in the field of bipolar disorder, and they often criticize the prescription habits of general practitioners, as the quote below illustrates:

> Interestingly, many fewer people being treated by bipolar disorder experts are on antidepressants:
> - Treated by community psychiatrists—80 percent of patients are on antidepressants
> - Treated by mood disorder clinics—50 percent of patients are on antidepressants

- Treated by specialty bipolar clinics—20 percent of patients are on antidepressants

So it would seem that the more specialized the care, the more professionals recognize the concerns over antidepressants. (Tracy, Breaking Bipolar, July 10, 2013)

As such views are expressed in posts where they provide the latest insights into a particular treatment, it would appear that these bloggers position themselves as more up to date than some medical professionals. Collins and Evans' (2002) conceptualization of expertise is based upon the idea that no contributory expert is equally competent in all areas pertaining to a particular domain. From this point of view, it remains open for debate whether these online contributions are attempts to fill relevant epistemic gaps or whether they represent interventions through which the bloggers challenge the authority and standing of medical professionals who are lower positioned than specialists and scientists, for instance.

This ambiguity is further exacerbated by the fact that such online comments are balanced by entries where Tracy and Fast warn readers about their lack of medical credentials and take up a complementary function to medical professionals. They try, for instance, to prevent people from quitting their medication when scandals related to pharmaceutical companies emerge. Fast even depicts herself (and people diagnosed) as useful allies, helping doctors identify dishonest claims made by pharmaceutical companies through their experiential knowledge of the effects and side effects of medications (Fast, Bipolar Happens!, October 16, 2016). Furthermore, multiple entries (Tracy, Breaking Bipolar, July 5, 2012) show that through their immersion in the community of medical professionals, these bloggers have also become familiar with the political economy of the pharmaceutical industry.

Another way in which they display their fluency in medical knowledge is by evaluating the merits of various studies and by distinguishing between medical information based on its source. In so doing, Tracy and Fast often clarify the status of the knowledge on bipolar disorder currently available and the inferences that can be made on it, as the following excerpt indicates:

It's time to get clear on what we really know about brain scans and #bipolar. It's so frustrating to read articles and studies about bipolar and brain imaging. At this time, there is NO brain image scan for the diagnosis of bipolar. Please do not pay someone who tells you that they can determine bipolar from an MRI or PET scan. It simply isn't true.

This is nascent science. One study shows some grey matter thinning in 3000 patients, another shows 'abnormal' activity in the amygdala and frontal lobes. There is nothing definitive and even if someone did find a change in the brain, without having a management plan that works, the information is just that… information. (Fast, Bipolar Happens!, July 18, 2018)

Fast performs interactional expertise by showing her familiarity with medical technology and terminology, and by being able to distinguish hopes and visions from the current relevance of brain scans in the diagnosis of bipolar disorder. Concerned about the quality of information that people diagnosed may acquire even from medical sources, Fast positions herself as a mediator, by using her own knowledge in order to correct erroneous assumptions and expectations. The bloggers also perform interactional expertise through their careful selection of the sources of information they use in their posts, as the excerpt below shows:

I'm pretty fussy about which medical and mental health resources I like, and which ones I don't. While there are many bipolar and mental health resources out there, I'm only interested in accurate *verifiable and reliable* sources of information on bipolar disorder and mental illness. (Tracy, Bipolar Burble, *Bipolar and Mental Health Resources,*[1] emphasis in the original)

Through their online posts, Tracy and Fast thus show that they have become fluent in the language of medical professionals and have therefore successfully developed interactional expertise.

---

[1] https://natashatracy.com/bipolar-and-mental-health-resources/. Accessed on May 13, 2016.

A Strong Media Presence

While important, having (access to) considerable technical skills and developing interactional expertise are not sufficient for these bloggers to become online expert mediators. To function as successful mediators between medical professionals and people diagnosed, Fast and Tracy not only require ample opportunities to perform interactional expertise, but they also need a strong media presence, to increase their public visibility and standing. The two bloggers have achieved this by developing close relations with mass media outlets. Tracy has often been interviewed and has participated in documentaries about bipolar disorder. In 2008, Fast hosted a weekly radio program, *The Julie Fast Show*, on KTRO in Portland, during which she had a number of "special guests," medical professionals or people diagnosed with various mental health conditions, who often wrote about their experiences and participated in advocacy actions. She is regularly interviewed on diverse mental health issues, such as pop artist Britney Spears' nervous breakdown and actress Carrie Fisher's death, and writes on mental health in magazines such as *People* and *US Weekly*. Fast was also the original consultant for the character played by Claire Danes, the main protagonist who suffered from bipolar disorder in the popular drama series *Homeland*. Fast and Tracy have also published books about their experiences with bipolar disorder, thereby further extending their reach. In 2016, Tracy wrote *Lost Marbles: Insights into My Life with Depression and Bipolar*. Fast is the author of five books, which have sold over 250,000 copies, four of which are "on the Amazon.com mood disorder bestselling book list" (Fast, Bipolar Happens!, 2016).

Through such activities, the bloggers also reach broader audiences than bipolar patients and their families, thereby contributing to how bipolar disorder and other related conditions are understood by the general public. As they become more familiar with other media, these bloggers can use their skills for more political purposes, as they may generate public sympathy, emphasize the urgency of particular pieces of legislation or treatment provisions, or put forward more complex images of life with bipolar disorder. In so doing, Tracy and Fast expand their mediation work beyond the more immediately responsive online medium, translating, synthesizing, bringing together, and refining different types of knowledge about bipolar disorder in formats in which interaction is more difficult, takes more time, and occurs more frequently away from the public. Yet, it is precisely through their ability to use different media and to retain a coherent image across them that these bloggers further increase their influence and standing.

That their standing goes beyond that of the average blogger is indicated by the numerous awards Tracy and Fast have received. Tracy received the Beatrice Stern Media Award and the #ErasingtheStigma Leadership Award and has been listed as the fourth Health Maker in the top ten online influencers in the area of mental health by Sharecare.com. She was also a speaker at the National Council on Mental Health and Addictions Conference and is hailed as one of the "heroic" figures of people diagnosed with bipolar disorder. Another indicator that her reach goes beyond the small circle of family and friends of regular illness bloggers is the fact that she has been a contributor on health platforms and a subject matter expert on bipolar disorder at Answers.com, all of which have millions of visitors. Fast received the Mental Health American Journalism award for the Best Mental Health Column in the US. Furthermore, the blogs Tracy and Fast have authored have been voted many times among the best bipolar blogs.

Whereas Fast and Tracy's activities across multiple media help them acquire greater audiences, the distinctions they received function as references or recommendations. Consequently, they can use their public visibility and standing as important resources to facilitate the development of more varied and substantial collaborations, not only with people diagnosed, but also with medical professionals. While this is an important characteristic of online expert mediators, in the next part of the analysis I use these insights to make a theoretical contribution, by expanding the notion of interactional expertise. I do so by arguing that interactional expertise has a stronger bi-directional nature than Collins and Evans assume and that the effects of the medium through which interactional expertise is performed need to be taken seriously.

Online Practices and Theoretical Implications for Interactional Expertise

Substantial Interactions and Bi-directionality

Bi-directionality refers to the ability of people endowed with interactional expertise to function as mediators between others with the same kind of contributory expertise as they and with individuals who have contributory expertise in the field where they hold interactional expertise. Whereas bi-directionality is an important aspect of interactional expertise, Collins and Evans do not sufficiently theorize it. For Collins and Evans (2002), interactional experts translate the scientific practices of contributory experts in one field for people with contributory expertise in another field, and shape the knowledge contributory experts produce by questioning some of their practices or by making them aware of other perspectives on an issue of interest. Thus, Collins and Evans see interactional experts as providing contributory experts with sources of inspiration. Whereas they see such exchanges as taking place in both conditions of symmetry and asymmetry, in the latter case, they only seem to conceive of one direction for the acquisition of interactional expertise, as I explain below.

Collins and Evans (2002) do not provide much information about the acquisition of interactional expertise in conditions of symmetry, but they suggest that it occurs between experts who may find themselves equally well positioned in order to productively contribute to the solution of a certain problem. In such conditions, Collins and Evans (2002) state that any of the two groups may absorb the expertise of the other one by developing interactional expertise. One may imagine such a situation occurring, for instance, as two different types of medical professionals are consulted for the treatment of a difficult case. Which one of the two specialists takes charge and oversees the patient's treatment is "arbitrary" from Collins and Evans' point of view, as long as one of the doctors has or develops interactional expertise into the other medical field, in order to be able to make informed decisions about the therapeutic approaches based on relevant insights from both medical fields. While in this example, the two contributory experts need to solve a common problem, Collins and Evans (2002) also give examples of situations where interactional expertise is developed by experts to address their own specific goals. For instance, they often invoke sociologists, who need to become fluent in the practice language of the scientific group they study, to be able to successfully conduct a sociological analysis. In such cases, however, Collins and Evans (2002, 2017) conceive of the development of interactional expertise as the responsibility of the group doing the study or needing to solve a specific problem.

Collins and Evans (2002) tie the development of interactional expertise under conditions of asymmetry to instances when this type of expertise is needed to facilitate the integration of a certain (sub)type of contributory expertise into another, broader, form of contributory expertise, with which the first is continuous, for the satisfactory resolution of a complex problem. They give examples both of situations when third parties are involved and of instances when the integration of one type of expertise into the other occurs without external involvement. In the first case, Collins and Evans (2002) mention that such absorption may be mediated by people who are not contributory experts in any of the two fields, but who hold interactional expertise in both. For instance, a sociologist may translate the knowledge and perspectives of a (smaller) group of unaccredited and less influential experts into a language that the accredited experts can understand, in order to appreciate and be able to use the insights of the unaccredited experts to solve a common problem.

When discussing the development of interactional expertise under conditions of asymmetry, Collins and Evans (2002) tend, however, to ascribe the task or capability of acquiring interactional expertise to the group of experts which are better positioned to solve a certain problem because of the epistemic authority, legitimacy, and other resources they already enjoy. Thus, they provide a new reading of Wynne's (1992) study on the relationship between scientists and the Cumbrian farmers in the aftermath of the Chernobyl disaster, where the scientists failed to recognize the contributory expertise of the farmers, who lacked official accreditation. Collins and Evans (2002:255) state that for the farmers' insights to be taken seriously, the latter "would *not* have had to engage in a symmetrical conversation" (emphasis in the original), but the scientists would have had to be willing to incorporate the former's insights by developing the relevant interactional expertise. Another example testifying to the same perspective is that of medical professionals becoming interactional experts on the lived experiences of their patients, which Collins et al. (2017) more recently invoked. Importantly, in Collins and Evans' (2002:256) view, "only the party with interactional expertise can take responsibility for combining the [contributory] expertises."

This argument suggests that under conditions of asymmetry, Collins and Evans believe the more influential party has the necessary resources to develop interactional expertise. I argue, however, that interactional expertise can not only develop in a bottom-up direction, whereby stakeholders who already enjoy epistemic authority in a given field expand their expertise by absorbing knowledge from unofficially recognized contributory experts in a (sub)field of interest, but it can also be acquired in what may seem like a top-down manner. Thus, people who have contributory expertise in a field but are not officially accredited can become fluent in the practice language of relevant epistemic groups, if they are endowed with other necessary resources. The acquisition of interactional expertise might this way contribute toward the development of more symmetric relationships between people who enjoy different standing due to the status of the field in which they have contributory expertise. As the description below will show, even under conditions of asymmetry, people endowed with interactional expertise can engage in exchanges that are more substantial than having interesting conversations with contributory experts, as Collins and Evans (2002) believe. Furthermore, whereas in determining the (a)symmetric character of an interaction, Collins and Evans seem to focus mainly on epistemic standing and authority as the determining factors, I argue that the availability of other resources may help balance such exchanges. More attention should therefore be paid to the type and quality of the interactions between interactional and contributory experts in different fields and to how different conditions or types of asymmetry may affect them. The exchanges of the bloggers studied here are revelatory in this sense.

One of the challenges encountered by researchers interested in collaborating with patients is to enable their contributions (Hewlett et al., 2006). This is an area where online expert mediators engage in mediation work, as they succeed to develop a space where their readers can articulate their experiences and negotiate how they position themselves in relation to their condition and the medical community. The bloggers educate people diagnosed about medical terminology and perspectives, so that the latter are better able to engage in collaborative projects with researchers. This is important, because not all bipolar patients may have the time and be in the physical and mental state necessary to grapple with medical terminology and research methodology. Moreover, Tracy and Fast may provide people diagnosed with the confidence that the insights they have are relevant and valuable, thus enabling them to interact with medical professionals with the assurance and determination necessary to move toward more equal exchanges. They may also help those interested in research participation to develop the patience and distance necessary to accept results, which may contradict their personal views.

Next to bipolar patients, the bloggers have constituted themselves as valuable allies for medical professionals who lack but need their insights derived from the lived experience with bipolar disorder for various aims. Thus, online expert mediators can assist medical professionals to acquire interactional expertise regarding the embodied experience of bipolar disorder, and thus help them develop a broader perspective about this condition and novel research ideas. By positioning themselves as representatives of their bipolar readers, the bloggers provide medical professionals with important information regarding the research directions people diagnosed with bipolar disorder would find relevant. In a context where medical expertise continues to be challenged, online expert mediators further serve the interests of the medical community by bestowing additional credibility upon the scientific approaches they champion.

The bloggers have also acquired sufficient medical knowledge and other relevant resources for medical professionals to agree to collaborate with them. Tracy noted that

> in my role I've been lucky enough to meet some really great professionals, some really great psychiatrists and researchers in their own right. And because I've gotten to know them through various acquaintances and through various things that I've done, if I want to do something that is scientific in nature, which I have done, then I can actually approach them

and say: "Look, I really have an interest in doing this. Do you have an interest in supporting this?" And we can work together to make it happen. (Tracy, March 29, 2021, online interview)

For instance, together with Prakash Masand, M.D., Tracy wrote an article published in 2014 in the medical journal *The Primary Care Companion for CNS Disorders*. Furthermore, in July 2016, she initiated a survey about patients' experiences concerning electroconvulsive therapy (ECT) on her personal blog:

> My name is Natasha Tracy and this ECT survey was my idea. I am running this survey with Dr. Prakash Masand [hyperlink provided], the psychiatrist behind the site Global Medical Education [hyperlink provided] which aims to educate others, particularly doctors, about medical issues such as those surrounding mental illness.
>
> For my part, I have bipolar disorder and have had ECT for bipolar depression. This has made me passionate about the subject as I see the extreme debate that goes on about this treatment online. (Tracy, Bipolar Burble, July 3, 2016)

While she is knowledgeable enough to come up with this idea and for an authoritative medical figure to collaborate with her, Tracy needs this partnership to legitimate her endeavor, since she lacks the apparently still necessary official accreditations.

Like Tracy, Fast has also used her blog to encourage people to participate in studies she champions:

> Can We Diagnose Bipolar Disorder Using Eye Images? (…)
> This is the question a new study from Souther [sic] Methodist University poses based off of my work on recognizing signs of mania in the eyes. Please visit the website and read more about this potently life changing study. What if we could see that we are manic through a physical sign even when our brain is telling us we are just fine? Think of the possibilities.
> Click here to read more about the SMU Mania in the Eyes Research Study. [hyperlink provided]

If you love my work, I would love your support of this project. Even one picture helps! (Fast, Bipolar Happens!, September 27, 2017)

Both excerpts suggest that one of the ways in which this new type of stakeholder can make themselves interesting for medical professionals to want to collaborate with them is by using their popularity among people diagnosed with bipolar disorder to encourage them to provide the data scientists need for research. While medical professionals acquire through such collaborations much needed data, the bloggers profit from the credibility and legitimacy of research findings obtained through collaborations with officially recognized experts, as Tracy notes

I don't have the credibility behind me in terms of getting published in a journal. So it's very important that I collaborate with someone who does, so that the results of something can be published in a way that not just people on my blog are going to see, but actually doctors are going to see, and doctors are going to respect. Because I can be the best writer in the world or the worst writer in the world … if I run a blog, doctors aren't necessarily going to pay attention to that whatsoever. It's understandable. But publishing something in a journal, that's going to get their attention. And I, just Natasha Tracy, can't really expect to do that very reasonably. (Tracy, March 29, 2021, online interview)

More such collaborations may develop in the future, given that the expertise of these bloggers about bipolar disorder has been publicly acknowledged by medical professionals. For instance, Ronald Pies, M.D., wrote about Tracy:

As a specialist in bipolar disorders, I can say that Natasha's understanding of this illness is more accurate and sophisticated than that of many physicians I have encountered over the past 30 years. But more than that: she shows uncommon wisdom and deep compassion, when it comes to discussing psychiatrists and psychiatry. (Pies, Psychiatric Times, May 24, 2012).

In her turn, Fast has co-authored the books *Take Charge of Bipolar Disorder: A 4-Step Plan for You and Your Loved Ones to Manage the Illness and Create Lasting Stability* (2004), *Loving Someone with Bipolar Disorder* (2004), and *Get It Done When You're Depressed* (2008) together with Dr. John Preston. He is now professor emeritus with Alliant International University in Sacramento, the author of 21 books, and the recipient of the "President's Award" from the Mental Health Association and of "Distinguished Contributions to Psychology Award" from the California Psychological Association. Fast is also claimed to "train pharmacists, psychiatric residents, social workers, alternative health care practitioners, general physicians, nurse practitioners, therapists and many more health care professionals on the topics of depression and bipolar disorder management" (Amazon, 2016). Reflecting on *The Health Cards Treatment System for Bipolar Disorder*, which she developed for people diagnosed with bipolar disorder and their family members, and which "works with or without medications," as she claims (Bipolar Happens!, 2016), Fast states: "I know that tens of thousands of my readers use the Health Cards daily… (…) Even my health care professionals use them!" (Fast, Bipolar Happens!, May 6, 2010). While using Fast's cards attests to an awareness by medical professionals that bipolar patients and their families may have needs which traditional medical approaches insufficiently address, it may also be a means for them to retain monopoly over medical knowledge at a time when other professionals challenge it. For the time being, however, both Fast and Tracy as well as the medical professionals they work with profit from forging alliances, and such substantial exchanges are characteristic for the activities of online expert mediators.

These bloggers are thus more than interesting and inspiring conversation partners for medical professionals. They are stakeholders that researchers want to collaborate with substantially, as they can facilitate the enrolment of a high number of study participants, and they can provide experiential knowledge and important insights into relevant areas for future research. The way for such partnerships has already been paved by patient organizations, but there have also been several substantial collaborations between researchers and particular individuals. Notable in this sense are the research activities of Portia Iversen (Iversen, 2007) and Sharon Terry (Terry & Boyd, 2001), who have directly contributed to the development of new therapeutic approaches for autism, and to the identification of the gene mutation causing pseudoxanthoma elasticum

(PXE), respectively. Yet, whereas Iversen and Terry had control over important resources as the leaders of two influential patient groups and were not themselves diagnosed with the conditions they studied, Tracy and Fast are bipolar patients and have managed to acquire the resources mentioned above individually, through their skillful use of the Internet.

Interactional Expertise and the Use of a Specific Medium

In their conceptualization of interactional expertise, Collins and Evans do not consider the effects of the medium through which interactional expertise is produced. I expand this notion by showing that the Internet has importantly shaped how Tracy and Fast have performed their interactional expertise. Studying how the Internet shapes the performance of interactional expertise is particularly important, since "in the context of the digital shift, the demarcation between certified experts and lay people is blurring" (Dickel & Franzen, 2016:3). This topic has generated a lot of interest among scholars in the field of science education and science communication, who have studied how the public responds to or engages with scientific knowledge provided via different media. Important in this sense is a study conducted by Shanahan (2010) on how scientific and personal expertise about health was expressed and discussed in the online comments section of a newspaper. Her study showed that even in peer-to-peer interactions, the most appreciated comments were those of contributors who claimed (some level of) scientific rather than personal expertise. Even though the online exchanges between the blog authors studied here and their readers may be conceived as peer-to-peer interactions due to the shared diagnosis of bipolar disorder and certain embodied experiences, there are important differences that need to be considered. Unlike the contributors scrutinized by Shanahan (2010), Tracy and Fast are individuals with a well-established public persona, who have to further demonstrate the interactional expertise displayed in their posts by (not) engaging with their readers' comments. While their audience may include contributory and interactional experts, an important difference from Shanahan is that such exchanges already take place in conditions of inequality, since as authors and owners, the bloggers speak to their readers, as some of the quotes provided above indicate. Shanahan's findings are nevertheless relevant, showing that online scientific expertise is not determined based on the invocation of credentials, but on one's ability to take up scientific practices, such as the provision of evidence and the citation of relevant sources, thereby revealing one's familiarity with the scientific norms and culture.

Such approaches were adopted by Tracy and Fast as a means to articulate and reinforce their online standing. For instance, comments from readers are used as opportunities to display their expertise by giving additional medical information and by correctly identifying specific interventions. Since people with experiential expertise display growing tendencies toward scientization in their contributions (Shanahan, 2010), these bloggers do not merely invoke scientific claims, but carefully select, apply, and interpret them. This is how Tracy reacts to a vague comment about a new test meant to determine the effectiveness of medical treatments for bipolar disorder: "I believe you're talking about the cytochrome P450 (CYP450) tests which I know are offered at the Mayo Clinic. (Also used in cancer treatment)" (Tracy, Breaking Bipolar, November 5, 2012). Thus, apart from having sufficient knowledge to understand what the contributor is referring to, Tracy also contextualizes the test, linking it to other medical disciplines. The bloggers further use their readers' comments as indicative of their informational needs and as sources of inspiration for some of their posts. From this perspective, comments help bloggers retain their popularity and influence by addressing topical issues.

Yet, the Internet also poses challenges to the display of interactional expertise, as the information they provide is open to the scrutiny of people with different levels of education, different views, and at different moments in time. To become and remain credible mediators, Tracy and Fast therefore need to show that the knowledge they share is authoritative while staying open to different perspectives. One way in which they manage such contradictory expectations is by using the Internet's multiplicity, giving different nuances to their messages on different platforms. They further use the asynchronous and selective character of comment exchanges to react advantageously to their readers' unexpected questions or reactions. Since Tracy and Fast are at liberty to choose when they react to comments, they can take the time to acquire more information or to work on a reply until it has a satisfactory shape. In the meantime, other readers may come to their "help," by sharing their knowledge and experiences. The bloggers' successful display of interactional expertise is also informed by the wise selection of instances when they interact with their readers. Thus, while they choose to intervene in situations where their knowledge, empathy, and relatability are emphasized, they remain silent in front of provocations which may alienate their audiences. Comments rules are another important instrument through which the bloggers may contain their readers' challenges and avoid controversy. For instance, initially Tracy did not allow commentators to provide the exact names and dosage combination of medicines. While this approach was meant to prevent readers from trying medicines without medical approval, it also weakened the epistemic claims and challenges they could bring against her.

The technology of blogs also enables Tracy and Fast to display their interactional expertise using images and hyperlinks. Their blog entries are often accompanied by images which either illustrate the main message of the post or bring an additional dimension to the information provided in writing. Depending on the topic, the bloggers choose for different ratios between written material and images. For instance, when discussing alternative ways of ensuring mood stability, Fast only writes a few lines but provides numerous images depicting relaxing activities. When the effects of particular medications are discussed, however, the written text dominates. At the same time, both bloggers provide videos of themselves on the blog, where they talk about certain experiences or advise their audiences. While it may be that their use of videos is informed by curiosity and by the desire to experiment with new technologies and opportunities available to update their blogs, such videos also serve to enhance the authenticity of their accounts, and to strengthen the bond between themselves and their readers. Through the use of video, the person behind the text of many posts, books, and magazine articles becomes a three-dimensional being, who moves and talks in particular ways, whose appearance may reveal the presence of bipolar disorder, or who may be the embodiment of its successful management.

Hyperlinks reveal important alliances as well as power relations. Both bloggers use them in order to show that the information they provide is based on reliable sources. They refer mainly to articles available in medical databases such as PubMed and Medscape or to posts by medical professionals on platforms where they collaborate. Tracy and Fast thus position themselves as trustworthy mediators between reliable sources of medical knowledge and interested audiences. Hyperlinks are also used by bloggers to emphasize their vast body of work. For instance, Tracy uses them to direct readers to her older posts. Interestingly, the bloggers generally refrain from using these affordances to share knowledge produced by other people lacking accreditations or to introduce their readers to projects initiated by "citizen scientists." This indicates that the high standing these bloggers enjoy is not due to a subversive use of the Internet, but rather due to their alliances with powerful stakeholders.

It is important to note that there are also significant differences between the ways in which Tracy and Fast use the Internet. Tracy's blog is highly interactive, having posts which acquire hundreds of comments, and she uses integrated approaches to increase the visibility of new posts. Thus, Tracy often uses Twitter and Facebook to notify readers about news on her blog, while Twitter updates are provided on her blog's main page. That interactivity is very important to her can also be derived from the fact that very popular blog posts and the posts with the most recent reactions are also listed on the first page, as you can see in Fig. 5.1, thereby guiding visitors on her page and encouraging them to engage in specific actions.

On Tracy's blog, the number of comments each post acquires is listed below the title and a hyperlink is provided, so that interested readers can directly access them rather than read the post. The hyperlink also draws attention to the comments visually, since it is provided in blue whereas the remainder of the information about a specific post is typed in black.

The number of comments available for the posts is not directly visible, but readers need to press an additional button to see them (Fig. 5.2), and the comment function is not available for all posts. Unlike Tracy, her posts generally receive a small number of comments, yet her blog continues to be voted among the best bipolar blogs currently available. To a certain extent, the limited interactivity on Fast's blog may be due to the fact that it developed as a continuation of a newsletter, so she may be accustomed to use the blog mainly to share information. Since many of

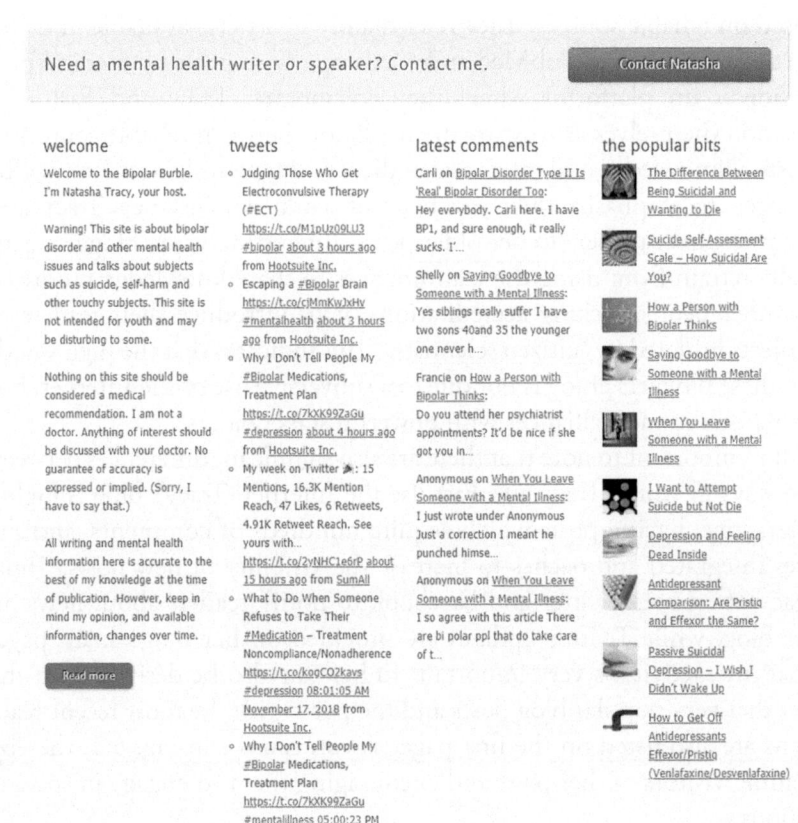

Fig. 5.1 Fragment from the first page of Natasha Tracy's blog, Bipolar Burble. Retrieved on January 8, 2019

her blog posts contain hyperlinks to her contributions in the online forum of *bp Magazine*, it may be that Fast prefers to have only one designated platform at a time for online interactions and to have ascribed this function to the forum. It may also be the case that she prefers personal correspondence with her readers, since she mentioned answering hundreds of letters per week at the time when she had just started circulating her newsletter, a habit which she may have preserved.

In general, both bloggers adapt the combination of medical and experiential knowledge, so that it is in line with the type of platform they contribute on, they react to comments strategically, and they are very

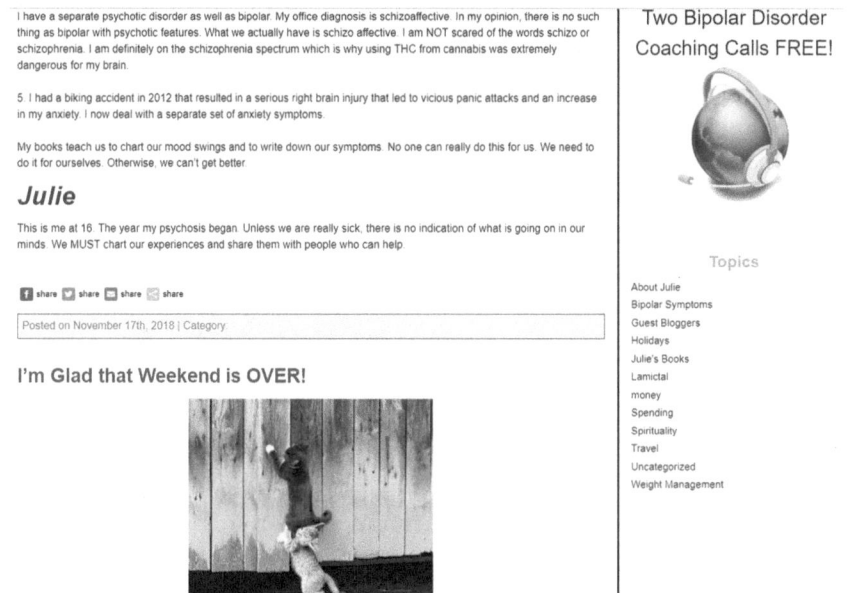

I have a separate psychotic disorder as well as bipolar. My office diagnosis is schizoaffective. In my opinion, there is no such thing as bipolar with psychotic features. What we actually have is schizo affective. I am NOT scared of the words schizo or schizophrenia. I am definitely on the schizophrenia spectrum which is why using THC from cannabis was extremely dangerous for my brain.

5. I had a biking accident in 2012 that resulted in a serious right brain injury that led to vicious panic attacks and an increase in my anxiety. I now deal with a separate set of anxiety symptoms.

My books teach us to chart our mood swings and to write down our symptoms. No one can really do this for us. We need to do it for ourselves. Otherwise, we can't get better.

Julie

This is me at 16. The year my psychosis began. Unless we are really sick, there is no indication of what is going on in our minds. We MUST chart our experiences and share them with people who can help.

share   share   share   share

Posted on November 17th, 2018 | Category:

I'm Glad that Weekend is OVER!

Two Bipolar Disorder Coaching Calls FREE!

Topics

About Julie
Bipolar Symptoms
Guest Bloggers
Holidays
Julie's Books
Lamictal
money
Spending
Spirituality
Travel
Uncategorized
Weight Management

Fig. 5.2 Fragment from the blog posts' overview on Julie A. Fast's blog, Bipolar Happens! Retrieved on November 5, 2018

careful in their use of hyperlinks. Thus, their display of interactional expertise is importantly shaped by their use of blog affordances.

Discussion

The bloggers discussed here can be seen as a particular and highly successful form of entrepreneurial selves (Petersen & Lupton, 1996). While this new type of stakeholder—online expert mediators—may fulfill a complementary or additional function to social movements, it also represents a move away from them and a focus upon exceptional patient figures, who have been able to use various resources and the opportunities and limitations the Internet has made available to become highly influential. This stakeholder category emerges thus at the intersection between a (mental) health condition, the acquisition of particular types of knowledge, and the use of a specific medium. By combining personal experiences with medical knowledge, Tracy and Fast have gone beyond the average illness blog, where one's personal experiences are conveyed in an intimate, diary-like fashion, and have come closer to issue-based blogs, where different types of information considered relevant about a particular topic are provided and discussed using arguments and multiple perspectives (O'Neil, 2005). The interactional expertise that they develop and articulate to various degrees has a strong bi-directionality, as they need to be fluent in the language of medical knowledge of bipolar disorder as well as to retain their experiential knowledge in a format which allows them to relate to readers diagnosed with bipolar disorder and their families. Thus, in their acquisition and articulation of interactional expertise, online expert mediators are reminiscent of journalists, who "develop different degrees of bipolar 'interactional expertise', specializing in interactions with their sources on the one hand and audiences on the other" (Reich, 2012:339). Furthermore, the online and offline activities of these bloggers foreground the importance of focusing on the multiple shifting identities that stakeholders can call upon in their development and performance of expertise. Their highly influential position was achieved through their ability to skillfully switch between their identity as individuals diagnosed with bipolar disorder, as successful blog owners, as representatives of many people diagnosed with bipolar disorder, and so on. I have taken up these insights in the conceptualization of expertise I put forward, where expertise is approached as a practical achievement realized through coordination and affective labor among stakeholders who occupy multiple and shifting positions within a complex ecosystem.

The rise of these stakeholders takes place in a context in which the informational and health imperatives require people to assume responsibility about their health (Kivits, 2013), yet the difficulties of living with a particular condition may lead them to prefer to follow someone else's lead (Lemire et al., 2008). Since the expertise of medical professionals has been challenged over the last few decades, many people diagnosed may seek to resolve this tension by following the advice of this new stakeholder type, by using such expert bloggers as arbiters. At the same time, the rise of this new stakeholder is also due to patients and their families requiring, apart from medical information, also encouragement and guidance. Nevertheless, these new stakeholders are also confronted with suspicion given the varying quality of the health information available online and the growing awareness that many public speakers and opinion setters represent particular groups of interest. To be successful, online expert mediators therefore need to convince their readers to develop different types of trust: they must trust the bloggers; they must trust certain online spaces or platforms; they must trust (at least) the branches of science the bloggers themselves rely upon (Harris et al., 2011). This also shows that the type of expertise these new stakeholders have acquired and perform online is a practical achievement, which they have realized by moving back and forth between relevant groups within the particular healthcare ecosystem in which they operate, by choosing to highlight particular aspects of their identity depending on the context and their goals, and by being caring but also careful toward other people and other types of knowledge.

Importantly, this chapter has indicated that the medium plays an important role in how interactional expertise is performed, thereby extending Collins and Evans' conceptualization of this notion. In so doing, it has also brought into relief some problematic aspects concerning the development of this new stakeholder category. While interactional expertise is necessary for this new type of stakeholdership, a strong medium is also needed. Developing interactional expertise has enabled Tracy and Fast to gain access and to develop close contacts with medical professionals, yet it is their online popularity, which has provided them with the resources necessary to engage in substantial exchanges with the latter. The Internet has therefore allowed them to convincingly position themselves as representatives of people diagnosed with bipolar disorder in their relations with medical scientists in a way that is reminiscent of the approach taken up by the American AIDS activists described by Epstein (1996). Epstein problematized the position "lay experts" occupy in relation to the "lay lay," highlighting that the acquisition of competence into a new type of knowledge impacts how one understands and relates to the other types of knowledge with which one is endowed as well as on one's relations to others. Thus, he warned that by "learning the language and culture of medical science" (Epstein, 1995:417) people diagnosed risk distancing themselves from other people diagnosed with the same condition, from their views and interests. From this perspective, the close collaborations the bloggers develop with medical professionals may lead to a further obfuscation of the differences in experience, interests, needs, and values that exist among the people diagnosed with bipolar disorder (Rowland et al., 2017) who follow their blogs.

While blogs have been acknowledged as technologies with a democratizing potential (Huovila & Saikkonen, 2016), the findings presented here show that online expert mediators acquire such high standing by developing close ties with "traditional" experts. Thus, rather than contributing to opening the field of scientific knowledge production to more people who lack official credentials, online expert mediators might inadvertently contribute to the refinement of existing hierarchies in the relations between medical professionals and patients. From this perspective, it is regrettable that the interactions between these bloggers and medical professionals occur most of the time offline or through private communication, so that it is not possible to observe how they negotiate participation in various projects and support for various initiatives. Since the bloggers' interactional expertise is limited to particular areas of medical knowledge on bipolar disorder and does not exclude personal preferences, online expert mediators also risk presenting their readers a skewed perspective on the use and effectiveness of the currently available forms of treatment. On a more positive note, the online expert mediators studied here may help bridge the digital divide when it comes to medical literacy by sharing medical knowledge in an accessible manner, by making people diagnosed and their families aware of the options at their disposal, and by helping them get in touch with support groups and other organizations. Having achieved a highly influential position, in the future they might harness their creativity and various skills to contribute in novel ways to the proliferation and diversification of collaborations between people diagnosed and medical professionals.

Ironically, whereas Fast started her online career after she moved to France, no French online bloggers enjoying similar standing to her and Tracy were identified. Since the use of the Internet for mental health–related purposes has been promoted by French authorities, as Chap. 3 has indicated, and since many people living in France have access to the

Internet, this is a rather puzzling finding. It is all the more surprising since the results described in Chap. 4 revealed that French online contributors were supporters of active forms of patienthood, and tried to actively manage their condition and to contribute to new knowledge about treatment effectiveness. The absence of this new type of stakeholder in France might be linked to particular social and cultural elements, which shape the use of the Internet and how people relate to their condition. While numerous French blogs on bipolar disorder could be identified, either they were read by few people or they had a very limited interactive character, receiving five comments or less for most posts. There were also blogs on bipolar disorder which enjoyed greater visibility, as they were authored occasionally on the online platforms of reputed French newspapers, such as *L'Avventura*, a caricature-based blog authored by Fiamma Luzzati for *Le Monde*, or *La Vie d'un Bipolaire*, authored by W. on the website of *L'Express*. Nevertheless, even in these cases, the level of interactivity was low. This might be informed by specific French cultural understandings and approaches to blogs, which conceive of them as online spaces where different types of information can be shared in a concise manner rather than as interactive platforms. This view is supported by the fact that even when famous medical professionals decided to share their views on blogs, these were not accompanied by a comment function. The fact that such medical professionals had become famous through their activities on radio and television suggests that rather than using the Internet to become influential, in France people use it as an additional medium, to reach more audiences or to convey the image of someone who is also up-to-date regarding online technologies.

Another explanation is that the absence of such influential individuals diagnosed with bipolar disorder or with any other condition, for that matter, may be due to the fact that the imperative for people to become active patients and assume responsibility for their health may have led in France to the development of entrepreneurial subjectivities that manifest themselves differently. An example in this sense is *Bipote*, the administrator and founder of *Le Forum des Bipotes* (LFB), mentioned in the previous chapter, who was also diagnosed with bipolar disorder. Even though as forum administrator, he had significant power and control, his position there was not as prominent and as influential as that of the bloggers studied here, despite his substantial knowledge about bipolar disorder. His preference for a forum rather than a blog may denote a preference for collective enterprises rather than individual approaches, and it may be that more people in France share this attitude.

The lack of this new type of stakeholder in the French landscape may also be informed by the fact that patient associations remain highly influential there, as they are active mediators between medical professionals, individuals diagnosed, and their families. As such, there may be little need among people diagnosed for this new type of stakeholdership to develop, whereas researchers and other official institutions may prefer to engage in collaborations with patient representatives they are familiar with and who are endowed with multiple types of knowledge and vast resources to mobilize people.

To conclude, the analysis of the activities of Tracy and Fast has provided important insights regarding some of the conditions necessary to become online expert mediators. Thus, next to an official diagnosis, people's health needs to be stable enough for them to engage in various activities requiring a lot of time and energy. They also need to be able to communicate in ways which can capture and retain the interest of different stakeholders. Furthermore, those interested need either to financially afford giving up their jobs to dedicate themselves to the development of blogs or to be willing to accept sponsorship or another form of payment, thereby running the risk of losing their social benefits. More research is needed to understand the ways in which other kinds of knowledge and online skills shape the acquisition and performance of interactional expertise, and into the differences and similarities concerning the mediation work undertaken by this new stakeholder category across different conditions. This chapter showed how individuals diagnosed with bipolar disorder responded to pronounced tendencies toward patient engagement by developing interactional expertise and used the Internet to become highly influential, thereby turning themselves into a new stakeholder category, what I called online expert mediators. The next chapter will describe a different response to such exhortations, as it focuses on solidarity and the development of a new type of community.

References

Adams, S. (2013). Maintaining the Collision of Accounts: Crowdsourcing Sites in Health Care as Brokers in the Co-Production of Pharmaceutical Knowledge. *Information, Communication & Society, 17*(6), 657–669.

Armstrong, D. (1995). The Rise of Surveillance Medicine. *Sociology of Health & Illness, 17*(3), 393–404.

Barak, A. (1999). Psychological Applications on the Internet: A Discipline on the Threshold of a New Millennium. *Applied & Preventive Psychology, 8*, 231–245.

Barak, A., & Grohol, J. (2011). Current and Future Trends in Internet-Supported Mental Health Interventions. *Journal of Technology in Human Services, 29*(3), 155–196.

Barak, A., Hen, L., Boniel-Nissim, M., & Shapira, N. (2008). A Comprehensive Review and a Meta-Analysis of the Effectiveness of Internet-Based Psychotherapeutic Interventions. *Journal of Technology in Human Services, 26*(2/4), 109–160.

Barbot, J. (2006). How to Build An "Active" Patient? The Work of AIDS Associations in France. *Social Science & Medicine, 62*, 538–551.

Barbot, J., & Dodier, N. (2002). Multiplicity in Scientific Medicine: The Experience of HIV-Positive Patients. *Science, Technology & Human Values, 27*, 404–440.

Barello, S., Graffigna, G., Vegni, E., & Bosio, A. (2014). The Challenges of Conceptualizing Patient Engagement in Health Care: A Lexicographic Literature Review. *Journal of Participatory Medicine, 6*(11), 1–15.

Barnes, M., & Shardlow, P. (1997). From Passive Recipient to Active Citizen: Participation in Mental Health User Groups. *Journal of Mental Health, 6*(3), 289–300.

Bottles, K. (2013). Health Hackers and Citizen Scientists Shake Up Medical Research. *Physician Executive Journal*, 88–90.

Brown, P. (1988). *The Transfer of Care: Psychiatric Deinstitutionalization and Its Aftermath*. Routledge Kegan & Paul.

Carlbring, P., & Andersson, G. (2006). Internet and Psychological Treatment. How Well Can They Be Combined? *Computers in Human Behavior, 22*, 545–553.

Collins, H., & Evans, R. (2002). The Third Wave of Science Studies. Studies of Expertise and Experience. *Social Studies of Science, 32*(2), 235–296.

Collins, H., & Evans, R. (2007). *Re-thinking Expertise*. The University of Chicago Press.

Collins, H., & Evans, R. (2015). Expertise Revisited, Part I — Interactional Expertise. *Studies in History and Philosophy of Science, 54*, 113–123.

Collins, H., Evans, R., Ribeiro, R., & Hall, M. (2006). Experiments with Interactional Expertise. *Studies in History and Philosophy of Science, 37*, 656–674.

Collins, H., Evans, R., & Weinel, M. (2017). Interactional Expertise. In U. Felt, R. Fouché, C. Miller, & L. Smith-Doerr (Eds.), *The Handbook of Science and Technology Studies* (4th ed., pp. 765–792). The MIT Press.

Crossley, M., & Crossley, N. (2001). "Patient" Voices, Social Movements and the Habitus: How Psychiatric Survivors "Speak Out". *Social Science & Medicine, 52*, 1477–1489.

Davidson, L. (2005). Recovery, Self Management and the Expert Patient-Changing the Culture of Mental Health from a UK Perspective. *Journal of Mental Health, 14*(1), 25–35.

De Boer, M., & Slatman, J. (2014). Blogging and Breast Cancer: Narrating One's Life, Body and Self on the Internet. *Women's Studies International Forum, 44*(1), 17–25.

Dickel, S., & Franzen, M. (2016). The "Problem of Extension" Revisited: New Modes of Digital Participation in Science. *Journal of Science Communication, 15*(1), 1–15.

Director, D. (2005). Using an Action Research Approach to Involving Service Users in The Assessment of Professional Competence. *European Journal of Social Work, 8*(2), 165–179.

Epstein, S. (1995). The Construction of Lay Expertise: AIDS Activism and the Forging of Credibility in the Reform of Clinical Trials. *Science, Technology & Human Values, 20*(4), 408–437.

Epstein, S. (1996). *Impure Science: AIDS, Activism, and the Politics of Knowledge*. University of California Press.

Fox, N., Ward, K., & O'Rourke, A. (2005). The "Expert Patient": Empowerment or Medical Dominance? The Case of Weight Loss, Pharmaceutical Drugs and the Internet. *Social Science & Medicine, 69*, 1299–1309.

Gillard, S., Simons, L., Turner, K., Lucock, M., & Edwards, C. (2012). Patient and Public Involvement in the Coproduction of Knowledge: Reflection on the Analysis of Qualitative Data in a Mental Health Study. *Qualitative Health Research, 22*(8), 1126–1137.

Goddiksen, M. (2014). Clarifying Interactional and Contributory Expertise. *Studies in History and Philosophy of Science, 47*, 111–117.

Godfrey, M., Callaghan, G., Johnson, L., & Waddington, E. (2003). *Supporting People: A Guide to User Involvement for Organizations Providing Housing Related Support Services*. Office of the Deputy Prime Minister.

Gowen, K., Deschaine, M., Gruttadara, D., & Markey, D. (2012). Young Adults with Mental Health Conditions and Social Networking Websites: Seeking Tools to Build Community. *Psychiatric Rehabilitation Journal, 35*(3), 245–250.

Grob, G. (2005). The Transformation of Mental Health Policy in Twentieth-Century America. In M. Gijswijt-Hofstra, H. Oosterhuis, J. Vijselaar, & H. Freeman (Eds.), *Psychiatry and Mental Health Care in the Twentieth-Century: Comparisons and Approaches* (pp. 141–161). Amsterdam University Press.

Harris, A., Wyatt, S., & Kelly, S. (2011). Conceptualizing Trust in Digital Environments. Health-e skepticism: Trust in the Age of the Internet. In: *A Decade in Internet Time: Symposium on the Dynamics of the Internet and Society* (OII-ICS Symposium), Oxford, UK, 21–24 September 2011, 1–11.

Heilferty, C. (2009). Toward A Theory of Online Communication in Illness: Concept Analysis of Illness Blogs. *Journal of Advanced Nursing, 65*(7), 1539–1547.

Hewlett, S., Wit, M., Richards, P., Quest, E., Hughes, R., Heiberg, T., & Kirwan, J. (2006). Patients and Professionals as Research Partners: Challenges, Practicalities, and Benefits. *Arthritis Care & Research, 55*(4), 676–680.

Hickey, G., & Kipping, C. (1998). Exploring the Concept of User Involvement in Mental Health Through a Participation Continuum. *Journal of Clinical Nursing, 7*, 83–88.

Hogg, C. (2009). *Citizens, Consumers and the NHS: Capturing Voices*. Palgrave Macmillan.

Huovila, J., & Saikkonen, S. (2016). Establishing Credibility, Constructing Understanding: The Epistemic Struggle Over Healthy Eating in the Finnish Dietetic Blogosphere. *Health, 20*(4), 383–400.

Iversen, P. (2007). *Strange Son: Two Mothers, Two Sons, and the Quest to Unlock the Hidden World of Autism*. Riverhead Books.

Kallinikos, J., & Tempini, N. (2014). Patient Data as Medical Facts: Social Media Practices as a Foundation for Medical Knowledge Creation. *Information Systems Research, 25*(4), 817–833.

Kemp, P. (2010). The Creative Involvement of Service Users in the Classroom. In J. Weinstein (Ed.), *Mental Health, Service User Involvement and Recovery* (pp. 15–29). Jessica Kingsley Publishers.

Kivits J (2013) E-Health and Renewed Sociological Approaches to Health and Illness. In Orton-Johnson K, Prior N (eds.) Digital Sociology. Critical Perspectives. Houndmills: Palgrave Macmillan, 213-226.

Klawiter, M. (1999). Racing for the Cure, Walking Women, and Toxic Touring: Mapping Cultures of Action within the Bay Area Terrain of Breast Cancer. *Social Problems, 46*(1), 104–126.

Kopelson, K. (2009). Writing Patients' Wrongs: The Rhetoric and Reality of Information Age Medicine. *Journal of Advanced Composition, 29*, 353–404.

Kraus, R., Stricker, G., & Speyer, C. (Eds.). (2010). *Online Counseling: A Handbook for Mental Health Professionals* (2nd ed.). Elsevier Academic Press.

Kushner, H. (2004). Competing Medical Cultures, Patient Support Groups, and the Construction of Tourette's Syndrome. In R. Packard, P. Brown, R. Berkelman, & H. Frumkin (Eds.), *Emerging Illnesses and Society: Negotiating the Public Health* (pp. 71–101). John Hopkins University Press.

Landzelius, K. (2006). Introduction: Patient Organization Movements and New Metamorphoses in Patienthood. *Social Science & Medicine, 62*(3), 529–537.

Latour, B. (2005). *Re-assembling the Social. An Introduction to Actor-Network Theory*. Oxford University Press.

Lemire, M., Sicotte, C., & Paré, G. (2008). Internet Use and The Logics of Personal Empowerment in Health. *Health Policy, 88*, 130–140.

Lerner, B. (2001). No Shrinking Violet: Rose Kushner and the Rise of American Breast Cancer Activism. *Western Journal of Medicine, 174*(5), 362.

Lucivero, F., & Prainsack, B. (2015). The Lifestylization of Healthcare? Consumer Genomics' and Mobile Health as Technologies for Healthy Lifestyle. *Applied & Translational Genomics, 4*, 44–49.

Lupton, D. (1995). *The Imperative of Health: Public Health and the Regulated Body*. Sage Publications.

Lupton, D. (2014). The Commodification of Patient Opinion: The Digital Patient Experience Economy in the Age of Big Data. *Sociology of Health & Illness, 36*(6), 856–869.

Marks, I., Cavanagh, K., & Gega, L. (2007). *Hands-On Help. Computer-Aided Psychotherapy*. Psychology Press.

Mazanderani, F., Locock, L., & Powell, J. (2012). Being Differently the Same: The Mediation of Identity Tensions in the Sharing of Illness Experiences. *Social Science & Medicine, 74*(4), 546–553.

McLean, A. (2000). From Ex-Patient Alternatives to Consumer Options: Consequences of Consumerism for Psychiatric Consumers and the Ex-Patient Movement. *International Journal of Health Services, 30*(4), 821–847.

Mulveen, R., & Hepworth, J. (2006). An Interpretative Phenomenological Analysis of Participation in a Pro-Anorexia Internet Site and Its Relationship with Disordered Eating. *Journal of Health Psychology, 11(2): 283,* 296.

Naslund, J., Aschbrenner, K., Marsch, L., McHugo, G., & Barteks, S. (2015). Crowdsourcing for Conducting Randomized Trials of Internet Delivered Interventions in People with Serious Mental Illness: A Systematic Review. *Contemporary Clinical Trials, 44,* 77–88.

Nettleton, S. (2004). The Emergence of E-scaped Medicine? *Sociology, 38*(4), 661–679.

Nicholas, J., Larsen, M., Proudfoot, J., & Christensen, H. (2015). Mobile Apps for Bipolar Disorder: A Systematic Review of Features and Content Quality. *Journal of Medical Internet Research, 17*(8), e198.

Novas, C. (2006). The Political Economy of Hope: Patients' Organizations, Science and Biovalue. *BioSocieties, 1,* 289–305.

O'Neil M (2005) Weblogs and Authority. *Selected Works.* University Paris IV Sorbonne. Accessed November 18, 2014, from https://works.bepress.com/mathieu_oneil/12/

Orsini, M., & Smith, M. (2010). Social Movements, Knowledge and Public Policy: The Case of Autism Activism in Canada and the US. *Critical Policy Studies, 4*(1), 38–57.

Petersen, A., & Lupton, D. (1996). *The New Public Health. Health and Self in the Age of Risk.* Sage.

Pickersgill, M. (2012). What is Psychiatry? Co-Producing Complexity in Mental Health. *Social Theory & Health, 10,* 328–347.

Plaisance, K., & Kennedy, E. (2014). A Pluralistic Approach to Interactional Expertise. *Studies in History and Philosophy of Science, 47,* 60–68.

Proudfoot, J. (2004). Computer-Based Treatment for Anxiety and Depression: Is It Feasible? Is It Effective? *Neuroscience and Behavioral Reviews, 28,* 353–363.

Rabeharisoa, V., Moreira, T., & Akrich, M. (2013). Evidence-based Activism: Patients' Organizations, Users' and Activist's Groups in Knowledge Society. *CSI Working Papers Series, 033,* 1–27.

Reich, Z. (2012). Journalism as Bipolar Interactional Expertise. *Communication Theory, 22,* 339–358.

Rose, N. (2007). *The Politics of Life Itself. Biomedicine, Power and Subjectivity in the Twenty-First Century.* Princeton University Press.

Rowland, P., McMillan, S., McGillicuddy, P., & Richards, J. (2017). What Is "The Patient Perspective" in Patient Engagement Programs? Implicit Logics and Parallels to Feminist Theories. *Health, 21*(1), 76–92.

Schaffer, R., Kuczynski, K., & Skinner, D. (2008). Producing Genetic Knowledge and Citizenship Through the Internet: Mothers, Pediatric Genetics, and Cybermedicine. *Sociology of Health and Illness, 30*(1), 145–159.

Shanahan, M. (2010). Changing the Meaning of Peer-To-Peer? Exploring Online Comment Spaces as Sites of Negotiated Expertise. *Journal of Science Communication, 9*(1), 1–13.

Sharon, T. (2017). Self-tracking for Health and the Quantified Self: Re-articulating Autonomy, Solidarity and Authenticity in an Age of Personalized Healthcare. *Philosophy & Technology, 30*(1), 93–121.

Smith, D. J., Griffiths, E., Poole, R., di Fiorio, A., Barnes, E., Kelly, M., Craddock, N., Hood, K., & Simpson, S. (2011). Beating Bipolar: Exploratory Trial of a Novel Internet-Based Psychoeducational Treatment for Bipolar Disorder. *Bipolar Disorders, 13,* 571–577.

Speed, E. (2006). Patients, Consumers, and Survivors: A Case Study of Mental Health Service User Discourses. *Social Science & Medicine, 62,* 28–38.

Taussig, K.-S., Rapp, R., & Heath, D. (2003). Flexible Eugenics: Technologies of the Self in the Age of Genetics. In A. Goodman et al. (Eds.), *Genetic Nature/Culture: Anthropology and Science Beyond the Two-Culture Divide* (pp. 58–76). University of California Press.

Terry, S., & Boyd, C. (2001). Researching the Biology of PXE: Partnering in the Process. *American Journal of Medical Genetics, 106,* 177–184.

Treichler, P. (1999). *How to Have Theory in an Epidemic: Cultural Chronicles of AIDS.* Duke University Press.

Turner, B. (1995). *Medical Power and Social Knowledge* (2nd ed.). Sage.

Tutton, R., & Prainsack, B. (2011). Enterprising or Altruistic Selves? Making Up Research Subjects in Genetics Research. *Sociology of Health & Illness, 33*(7), 1081–1095.

Wathen, N., Wyatt, S., & Harris, R. (Eds.). (2008). *Mediating Health Information: The Go-Betweens in a Changing Socio-Technical Landscape.* Palgrave Macmillan.

Whitley, R. (2012). The Antipsychiatry Movement: Dead, Diminishing, or Developing? *Psychiatric Services, 63*(10), 1039–1041.

Wyatt, S., Harris, A., Adams, S., & Kelly, S. (2013). Illness Online: Self-Reported Data and Questions of Trust in Medical and Social Research. *Theory, Culture & Society, 30*(4), 131–150.

Wynne, B. (1992). Misunderstood Misunderstanding: Social Identities and Public Uptake of Science. *Public Understanding of Science, 1*, 281–304.

Ybarra, M., & Eaton, W. (2005). Internet-Based Mental Health Interventions. *Mental Health Services Research, 7*(2), 75–87.

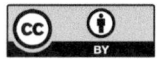

6

Digital Biocommunities: Solidarity and Lay Expertise About Bipolar Disorder

I had already taken the anxiolytics…

But I've managed to ask someone to help me on a forum because I couldn't take it anymore. Someone reacted and we're talking via private messages. I think this will help me a bit. Thanks. (*Derek21*, March 18, 2013)

Through their online activities, people diagnosed with bipolar disorder often engage in solidaristic behaviors, providing help and support to similar others in need, as the quote above illustrates. This draws attention to another important aspect of expertise, which is not only shaped by the means through which it is acquired and performed and by the goals it aims to achieve, but also by the values that motivate and support such processes. In recent years, expertise about bipolar disorder has been shaped by the rise of personalized and precision medicine (Evers, 2009; Ozomaro et al., 2013; Shin et al., 2016), which many believe will lead to highly individualized approaches to health and will thus have important moral consequences. Whereas autonomy has featured prominently in these debates, in recent years scholars have started to investigate how personalized and precision medicine might affect solidaristic practices. In so doing, influential commentators have challenged the dominant belief

© The Author(s) 2023
C. Egher, *Digital Healthcare and Expertise*, Health, Technology and Society,
https://doi.org/10.1007/978-981-16-9178-2_6

that these approaches would necessarily lead to radical forms of individualism, arguing, instead, that they could also prompt solidaristic approaches to healthcare (Prainsack & Buyx, 2017). In this chapter, I join this group of researchers by studying the tensions between the appeals to solidarity and individualization in mental healthcare triggered by personalized and precision medicine and by considering how these tensions are taken up and reflected in the online exchanges of American and French contributors diagnosed with bipolar disorder. In so doing, I engage in the exploration of the one remaining aspect of the conceptualization of expertise that I put forward in this book, namely its collective nature and the role of affective labor. Based on the analysis of the empirical materials, I argue that solidaristic practices underlie numerous online interactions among people diagnosed with bipolar disorder, thereby contributing to the development of a new type of collectivity—what I have called "digital biocommunities"—and promoting the development of lay expertise.

The Individualization of Healthcare: Solidarity Under Threat

The rise of personalized and precision medicine has taken place in a context marked by the demise of national welfare systems and by the growing dominance of neoliberal tendencies, which have introduced a market logic in the provision of healthcare and have focused on individual empowerment as a means to achieve collective well-being. Personalized and precision medicine has been fueled by insights from genomics and related fields and has profited from the availability and accessibility of a great number of online applications through which people can keep track of their health. Thus, health-related data have been expanded under precision medicine (Hedgecoe, 2004) to include a vast array of elements (Hogle, 2016; Weber et al., 2014), and individuals have been encouraged to engage in the self-tracking of a growing number of biological, environmental, and lifestyle elements (Lupton, 2018; Prainsack, 2017). While such practices address individuals as autonomous and self-interested beings, even in their most narrow or radical understanding, personalized and precision medicine relies on collectives for the comparison and interpretation of data. This renders the relationship between autonomy and solidarity at the same time important and problematic for researchers and policy makers alike. A good illustration in this sense comes from the Precision Medicine Initiative, whose name—All of Us—conveys a vision of healthcare meant to bring collective benefits, yet on whose website individual readers are interpellated by being told that "the future of health begins with you" (June, 2018). While for proponents of the Precision Medicine Initiative, individual autonomy appears to be needed to achieve solidarity, in France solidarity seems to be the means through which individual autonomy can be achieved, as the French version of the name of the National Fund for Solidarity and Autonomy (*La Caisse Nationale de Solidarité Pour L'Autonomie*[1]) suggests.

How the individualizing tendencies underlying personalized and precision medicine affect solidarity has also been the object of vigorous debates among scholars. Supporters have welcomed these tendencies as leading to better and more efficient ways to provide healthcare, which they claimed would ultimately benefit both the individual *and* society at large. Thus, by tailoring clinical investigations and therapeutic approaches to the specific needs and circumstances of every person (Wium-Anderesen et al., 2017), people would be spared unnecessary tests or therapeutic approaches less likely to be successful. This would enable the more effective attribution of funds in healthcare, thereby addressing and redressing a state of precarity triggered by a growing number of people diagnosed with (mental) health conditions and insufficient funds. Proponents of personalized and precision medicine have also invoked the language of empowerment, arguing that the widespread adoption of digital technologies and self-tracking enable people to gain more knowledge and control over their health (Knoppers & Chadwick, 2005; Steinhubl et al., 2013). In turn, this could contribute to the democratization of the relations between individuals and medical professionals or even to a hierarchical reversal thereof, as titles such as "Patient-Driven Health Care Models" (Swan, 2009) or *The Patient Will See You Now* (Topol, 2015) suggest.

---

[1] This institution was established in 2005 to distribute and oversee the national provision of financial help and assistance to people with disabilities and the elderly.

In contrast, critics have argued that by addressing individuals as unique from certain points of view, people may end up focusing more on what distinguishes them from others rather than on what binds them together, which may lead to "radical" differences. According to Dickenson (2013), such approaches could bring about a shift from "We Medicine" to "Me Medicine," a concern which is eloquently echoed by Prainsack and Buyx (2017:127):

> Because every patient is different, as this new version of personalized medi-cine assumes, their health and their diseases are different as well: individual differences in our genetic makeup, in our gene expression, in the microor-ganisms inhabiting our guts and bodies, in our lifestyles, diets and so forth render each of us, as well as our physiologies and pathologies, a unique expression of a particular state of health and disease in any given moment in time. (Prainsack & Buyx, 2017:127)

These approaches thus threaten solidarity and may lead to new forms of inequality and discrimination (Prainsack & Buyx, 2012), as people engaging in seemingly preventable individual behaviors, such as smoking or the consumption of sugar and fats, may be required to pay higher insurance rates, and/or may be denied access to some medical treatment and social provisions. These critics warn this way that individual freedom and responsibility can be invoked in such instances to mask systemic forms of economic and social inequality, and may even help to perpetuate them. Challenging what they consider to be the "tyranny of autonomy" (Foster, 2009) in Western healthcare and the understanding of individu-als as autonomous, rational, self-interested beings, such commentators (Baylis et al., 2008; Prainsack & Buyx, 2012) have argued instead in favor of a relational approach. From this point of view, individual identi-ties, values, needs, and perspectives are not dictated by self-interest alone, but importantly shaped by the other people in one's life and by the socio-political context in which one lives. There are indications that such per-spectives are supported by practices on the ground, as exemplified by the shift from "The Quantified Self" to "The Quantified Us" (Lupton, 2016) among proponents of health endeavors generally thought to be highly individualistic and individualizing, and by empirical studies that have identified solidaristic practices at the heart of self-tracking (Sharon, 2017).

Since I have argued that expertise is a collective notion, requiring the concerted efforts of numerous stakeholders, the expectation of "radical" individualization in healthcare raised important questions about its future and the new shapes that it may take. This was particularly the case for lay expertise, a collective notion whose meaning and relevance are rendered uncertain in a healthcare context marked by a focus on individual differences. The data used in this chapter were therefore initially approached with the expectation of encountering numerous instances confirming the idea that individual needs, preferences, and approaches in mental healthcare have become dominant to the detriment of more collective challenges and concerns. Yet, on many blogs and fora people diagnosed with bipolar disorder continued to seek to understand their condition collectively and displayed substantial concern for others. For instance, they tried to make sense of the symptoms they experienced by placing them in the broader context of their lives, by considering how their behaviors affected their families, friends, and colleagues, and by comparing their experiences with those of others with the same diagnosis. It thus became obvious that solidarity is a value that online contributors diagnosed with bipolar disorder perform online, which shifted the analytical focus onto its relation to lay expertise, thereby turning this chapter into a contribution to calls made by scholars to study how values manifest themselves in practice (Swierstra, 2013; van de Werff, 2018).

The Meaning of Solidarity

Despite solidarity's re-appearance in debates about health policy, the meaning of this concept remains evasive. While it is often defined as "the glue that keeps people together" (Komter, 2005:2), different perspectives have been put forward to explain how such social cohesion is achieved. Thus, some scholars approach solidarity as a particular set of feelings and emotions (Mayhew, 1971), as moral (Etzioni, 1988) and "affective ties" (Parsons, 1952:157) which inform people's commitment to others. In such cases, solidarity is intertwined with the human capacity to experience and express sympathy, care, and concern for people in their immediate surroundings. It is thus thought to spring into being rather automatically, informed by common attachments (instead of rational considerations) among a relatively small number of people. Others understand solidarity as a characteristic of groups and societies (Durkheim, 1964; Weber, 1947), regulating the interactions between the individual and the community (Bayertz, 1998), and potentially furthering the common good. Van Oorschot and Komter noted in this sense that "[t]he main source of solidarity is a mutual sharing of each other's fate" (1998, 8), thereby largely conceiving of solidarity as a result of rational choices and calculations (Hechter, 1987), of the acknowledgment of "shared identity" and "shared utility" (Van Oorschot & Komter, 1998). Yet other scholars approach solidarity as a moral, universal, "inclusive" ideal (Dean, 1995), prescribing specific sets of orientations and behaviors which people should take up in order to increase social bonds in the heterogeneous societies we currently live in.

The study of solidarity in this chapter is based, however, on the conceptualization put forward by Prainsack and Buyx (2012, 2017), which has the advantage of being concrete and practice-oriented. In their view (2012:346), "[s]olidarity signifies shared practices reflecting a collective commitment to carry 'costs' (financial, social, emotional, or otherwise) to assist others," and this conceptualization is underpinned by three important elements. First, it relies upon a relational understanding of personhood, as these scholars see the individuals' concerns, values, and preferences as emerging in interaction with those surrounding them and as shaped by the socio-cultural environment in which they find themselves. This allows for solidarity to be distinguished from altruism, as people are approached as simultaneously self-interested and concerned for the well-being of others. Second, solidarity is based upon the recognition of a relevant similarity, upon people's acknowledgment that they share a commonality with others in respect of interest. This makes it possible to distinguish it from charity, as solidaristic practices are understood to emerge among individuals or groups in symmetrical relations to each other in regard to the similarity that is relevant in a given context. Third, while feelings and emotions may play an important role in its development, solidarity is something that is done, performed. It is manifested through "enacted commitments" (Prainsack & Buyx, 2017:42), which may vary in scope and impact, ranging from a document or piece of policy to individual actions undertaken by private citizens. Attention to these three dimensions made it possible to study the provision of online texts as informed by solidarity and to focus on how online contributors diagnosed with bipolar disorder relate to or distinguish themselves from others rather than approach them as a homogeneous group. As this involves inclusions and exclusions, this conceptualization also has the advantage of precluding an approach to solidarity as something exclusively positive (Dean, 1995) and encourages a focus on how the affordances of online platforms may be implicated in such practices.

Solidarity and Idioms of Practice

In studying how solidarity relates to lay expertise online, I build upon multiple studies which have shown that a common diagnosis (Epstein, 2007; Rabeharisoa & Callon, 2002) and similarities in one's genetic profile and potential health risks facilitate the formation of collectives (Rabeharisoa et al., 2013) and can even contribute to "genomic solidarity" (Van Hoyweghen & Rebert, 2012). The analysis is particularly indebted to Rabinow's (1996) view that developments in genetics have led to the emergence of biosociality; that is, they have enabled the formation of new group and individual identities based on genetic and molecular insights. While new types of knowledge transform the ways in which people understand their condition and relate to others, online interactions are importantly shaped by the digital technologies they use, by the affordances of the social media where they seek and provide information. Thus "its [the internet's] interactivity and the interaction it allows for can facilitate the formation of specific points of view and new ways of articulating individual experience to collective positions" (Akrich et al., 2008:2). Online exchanges may therefore contribute to "fostering community and mutual support, and negotiating medical relationships" (Sosnowy, 2014:325). They may also prompt transformations in the very meaning and practice of sociality (van Dijck, 2013), as people figure out what aspects of a technology they use and how they use it in practice, by tinkering with it as they interact with others. Thus, not only do people use such technologies for social activities, but their very use is social, in that people "develop their beliefs about media and ways of using media within *idioms of practice*" (Gershon, 2010: loc 117). According to Gershon, "[i]dioms of practice point to how people have implicit and explicit intuitions about using different technologies, which they have developed with their friends, family members, and coworkers" (ibid.) and which "emerge out of collective discussions and shared practices" (ibid.).

The concept of idiom of practice underlines the multiple meanings that a technology can have, depending on its users and on the context of their engagement with it, on the ways in which those around them use it, and on the prevailing social norms and values that delineate what it should and should not be used for. In this sense, Gershon describes how the development of social media led to the development of various idioms of practice regarding acceptable forms of breakup. While some people considered breaking up via an e-mail a more acceptable approach, because it was more personal and private, others found that it resembled too much a monologue, and preferred being notified about such an occurrence on social media, where turn-taking could unfold faster and dynamic exchanges could easily occur. While in the early days of a technology, multiple idioms of practice can exist, in time certain practices may "solidify," as some uses become widespread in specific contexts. The analysis described in this chapter is based upon a theoretical framework where this concept is combined with the understanding of solidarity developed by Prainsack and Buyx (2017). This framework allowed for a better understanding of the roles that online platforms and their affordances play in the performance of this value, of the new forms of sociality that can thus be developed, and of how they relate to lay expertise.

Lay Expertise and Affective Labor

Lay expertise is typically developed as people diagnosed become better informed about the medical knowledge available about their condition, by learning to interpret their own embodied experiences in light of this knowledge and by engaging in various tinkering practices to better manage their symptoms in their daily lives. While acquiring medical knowledge is an activity that in theory one may conduct individually, the other processes at the heart of lay expertise generally require multiple social interactions, as people diagnosed encounter others with the same condition and start making sense of their experiences by comparing symptoms, treatment reactions, and life circumstances. Importantly, lay expertise is developed in conditions where people who are brought together by virtue of the same diagnosis come to experience feelings of trust, care, and concern for each other. This means that such processes are importantly underpinned by affective practices, by the various strategies through which people diagnosed manage their affects and seek to produce specific affects in those they interact with. Nevertheless, previous studies on lay expertise have mainly focused on the epistemic processes through which people diagnosed become very knowledgeable about their condition, and have generally neglected the affective practices, which support the processes of knowledge acquisition, exchange, and development. While such a lack of attention may be informed by the age-old dichotomy between ratio and affect, it is regrettable in a context where scholars have highlighted the epistemic value of emotions (Nussbaum, 2003). This is especially relevant in regard to online practices, as growing calls have been made to acknowledge them not only as communicative activities, but also as forms of labor, through which particular identities are claimed and networks are developed (Clough, 2008; McCosker, 2018; McCosker & Darcy, 2013).

To determine the role affective practices can play in the development of lay expertise online, it is important to understand how emotions have come to be associated with the sphere of labor. Psychologists have played an important role in this sense, as in the first decades of the twentieth century they highlighted the relevance of emotions for professional practices through their engagements with the army and corporations (Illouz, 2008). Thus, during the First World War, intelligence tests were developed, followed in the decades thereafter by personality tests and experiments on corporate productivity, which came to be increasingly applied in personnel recruitment and management (Lussier, 2018). Under the influence of mental healthcare professionals, the ability to control one's emotions and to manage those of others became the mark of rational and self-interested individuals and started to be seen as important competences, which could significantly further one's professional career (Illouz, 2008). As Hochschild (2012) showed in here studies on emotional labor, this trend has become all the more pronounced with the rise of the service economy, as the display of particular emotions is now integral part of various jobs. Work on and through emotions has not been reserved, however, only to the professional realm, but has also become integral to the development and management of the successful self in the realm of private life (Illouz, 2008). Illouz (2018:148) importantly remarked in this sense that "the growing focus on emotions in the psy-industries and their rising economic value in corporations and consumer culture (...) are intertwined with the rising cultural value of emotions in the constitution of self-identity, social relations and well-being." Writing and reading have been at the core of such developments, as they allowed individuals to decontextualize and fix what had hitherto been transient emotions, to reflect upon them, and, in so doing, to manage them. This is important for the analysis described in this chapter, because while such practices have generally been reserved for private diaries, online platforms allow these days for "networked public intimacy" (Kitzman, 2004), facilitating new approaches for online contributors to manage their selves and to lay claims to particular identities online.

Since online exchanges involve not only the management of one's emotions, but also those of others, the concept of affective labor is used to study how affective practices contribute to the development of lay expertise. Affective labor is understood as "labor that produces or manipulates affects such as feelings of ease, well-being, satisfaction, excitement, or passion" (Hardt & Negri, 2004:108), which take place at a pre-visceral stage of experience. Particularly relevant here is Hardt's (1999:89) view that affective labor is indicative of "processes whereby our laboring practices produce collective subjectivities, produce sociality, and ultimately produce society itself." This perspective allows me to focus on the personal and social value their online engagements may have for people diagnosed with bipolar disorder. Whereas a growing amount of value is nowadays generated from the cognition, communication, affect, and the immaterial actions of online "prosumers," the debate among scholars about the role of immaterial labor in digital media economics is still ongoing. Thus, Hardt and Negri (2004) join many others who have criticized users' engagement with digital technologies as a form of free labor (Lupton, 2014; Mitchell & Waldby, 2010; Terranova, 2000; Waldby & Cooper, 2008). More recently, however, a number of scholars (Andersson, 2017; Kneese, 2017; McCosker & Darcy, 2013) have shown that other forms of value or gratification that users of digital technologies may derive by engaging in immaterial labor need to be considered. This chapter builds upon the views of this latter group of researchers, as I argue that affective practices are an important, even though tacit, element of lay expertise, shaping it both directly and indirectly, through the collectives it supports into being.

The data underlying this analysis were collected from one French forum, *Troubles Bipolaires*, hosted on the online platform *Doctissimo*, and from one American forum, *bp Hope*. Two threads were selected from the first two pages of thread titles on the *Troubles Bipolaires*, which means that they had been among the most recently contributed to when the selection occurred. They were initiated in 2013 and 2014, respectively, and by February 20, 2018, one had gathered 1829 replies and the other 17,102. Fifteen threads from the *bp Hope* forum which had received at least 30 comments were selected. This selection criterion was determined by the need for numerous interactions in order to study the development of community. There is a considerable difference between the number of interactions studied on the French forum, which were also atypical for *Troubles Bipolaires*, and the ones on the American forum. Nevertheless, I decided to compare the two, in order to understand whether there was something specific about sociality on these two threads and whether the content, the contributors, and/or particular uses of online affordances explained this difference. While Chap. 4 focused on the treatment experiences of people diagnosed with bipolar disorder, for this chapter data were collected about two other important aspects in their lives—the lived experiences of the symptoms of this condition and personal and social life with/despite bipolar disorder. The data were analyzed using thematic analysis combined with approaches derived from conversation analysis, thus following in the footsteps of researchers who approach online interactions as forms of naturally occurring exchanges, given that they resemble offline dialogue in terms of turn-taking, action, and reaction (Armstrong et al., 2012; Kaufman & Whitehead, 2016).

Solidarity About Bipolar Disorder Online

Relevant Similarities

Online contributors were initially brought together on the fora studied by one important similarity: they had all been diagnosed with bipolar disorder. Behind this rather obvious commonality, many other similarities were conflated, such as a similar orientation toward bipolar disorder and similar approaches in trying to make sense of it and to address it effectively. Thus, long-lasting interactions developed among people who understood bipolar disorder as a biological condition, determined by genetic and neurological factors, and which could be managed through medication. This shared perspective was apparent, for instance, among online contributors who joked about not having children to prevent the transmission of their "bipolar genes," or referred to neural activity and faulty circuits in their brain to explain some of their behaviors.

Another commonality online contributors shared was the difficulty to narrow down the meaning and influence of bipolar disorder on other aspects of their health. For instance, while in terrible pain because of trigeminal neuralgia, a chronic pain condition that affects the trigeminal nerve, *Sylvana* confessed to feeling uncertain regarding the source of her pain. Since none of the procedures undertaken had been very successful, she had started doubting whether the pain she was experiencing was solely caused by the trigeminal nerve or whether her diagnosis of bipolar disorder also played a role, either by rendering her more sensitive to the experience of pain or more resistant to the effects of the medications prescribed. In a similar vein, *elaine43*, a contributor on the forum *bp Hope*, confessed to being uncertain whether the loss of memory she was experiencing was due to aging, hormonal changes induced by the menopause, neurological changes bipolar disorder had produced in her brain, or the long-term effect of the medications she had taken for its management. Such common uncertainties were often underlined by similarities in certain aspects of identity, such as age, gender, and level of education.

Online contributors identified additional similarities in the form that certain symptoms took for them or in the adjustments they required, such as the adaptation to a new location while on holiday, as the exchange below illustrates:

> Whether I go far away or not, it's the same. Once I have my bearings, it's ok, but I need to get used to the place.
> Sometimes this only happens late .... (georgette393, August 20, 2015)
> *
> Same here, but that's why I often go to places I know. The adaptation can take long for me ... Decidedly the bipos [people diagnosed with bipolar disorder] really tend to function the same way .... (+Vie, August 20, 2015)

The identification of such commonalities contributed to the contributors' feeling part of a community to such an extent that it prompted some of them to make inferences about all people diagnosed with this condition, as +*Vie*'s comment suggests.

The development of a shared idiom of practice further assisted online contributors to identify commonalities. For instance, frequent contributors on one of the *Troubles Bipolaires* threads developed the habit of sharing and updating elaborate personal descriptions on a separate location on the forum. This approach helped them discover similarities in terms of family circumstances, favorite pets, or places where they had lived. It also had the disadvantage, however, of rendering one's newcomer status more obvious, when online contributors did not use these distinct spaces on the forum as was customary. On *bp Hope*, the discovery of additional commonalities was assisted through the development of threads with a playful, socially informative character, such as "where were you when..." or "Sharing quotations." Next to the structured provision of such personal information, online contributors could identify similarities based on their profile photos, their motto, or online signatures, which conveyed through words and/or images their interests, hobbies, or political views.

Performing Solidarity

Having identified such similarities, online contributors performed solidarity by sharing personal strategies to better manage bipolar disorder in daily life, by informing others about the results of their self-experiments, and by creating a safe environment where concerns, preferences, and challenges could be expressed. The following exchange is illustrative in this sense:

> The part about psychosis resonates with me. People don't understand it and are frightened by it. I find that I can't talk about it with my loves ones because it just creates more worry. It's the most isolating part of my illness.
>
> I would add thoughts of self harm to the list. We all deal with it but it's not something we can talk about. (*beyondblue*, March 7, 2015)
> **1 user thanked author for this post: Mary**
> *
>
> Beyondblue,
> Self harm does seem to be a taboo subject, even on here. I understand the trigger it is for most but I think it's important to admit when those feelings are breathing over our shoulders. Not only for our own well being but so others know they are not alone.
> MO (*midnightowl*, March 7, 2015)

beyondblue's comment shows that he feels comfortable enough to accept the thread initiator's invitation to contribute to a list of less-talked-about symptoms experienced by people diagnosed with bipolar disorder. The first paragraph is important because it highlights the relational way in which this contributor experiences his condition as well as the affective labor he performs, as he takes into account the impact certain topics may have on his family and acts accordingly. The contrast between such avoidance behaviors toward one's family and the openness of one's online contributions highlights the important social function fulfilled by online platforms. The switch from "I" to "we" in the second paragraph indicates that *beyondblue* feels solidarity with the other online contributors based on a common, even though rather taboo, symptom.

midnightowl's reply to *beyondblue* confirms the solidaristic ethos underlying such sharing practices, as she encourages him to continue to talk about self-harm as a form of support for others. While she does not dwell upon it, *midnightowl* acknowledges that such sharing practices also further the well-being of the contributor, which supports the view put forward by Prainsack and Buyx (2017) that people act simultaneously out of self-interest and concern for others when engaging in solidaristic behaviors. Even though it is a light form of participation, *Mary's* appreciation of *beyondblue's* comment suggests that the online affordances on the forum ensured a minimal degree of reciprocity among information providers and information seekers and thus contributed to the development of relationships.

Online contributors also performed solidarity by putting time and effort into identifying reliable sources of information for those with whom they frequently interacted. As *Sylvana* was worried about a surgical procedure she was due to undergo, online contributors answered her invitation to help:

> you make me think that I should look for a very specific forum for "people in my case".
>
> if one of you is willing to do a search for me, I'm interested. (*Sylvana*, April 13, 2015)
> *
> so....
> on docti [N.B.link provided]
> next
> a discussion on vulgaris [N.B.link provided]
> then
> a forum [N.B.link provided]
> and afterwards
> a positive testimony [N.B.link provided]
> That done, you'll still need to look around...
> Right now I got to go pick up my son.... (*Rianne*, April 13, 2015)

Sylvana's first sentence highlights the tendency among online contributors to seek interactions with others with whom they share relevant similarities, and indicates that individuals may be simultaneously members of multiple online communities, where they focus on different issues of interest. *Rianne's* reply makes it obvious that she invests time in the context of a busy schedule and uses her online experience and personal knowledge of *Sylvana* to identify online sources of information that she believes would be of help to her online friend. The small description

Rianne provides about the online platforms she selected suggests that for these online contributors, interactive online platforms where people can engage in dialogue are important sources of lay expertise, which they find useful in case of doubt or anxiety. The list can also be understood as the result of affective labor, as *Rianne* keeps her list short and easily legible, and includes in it a positive testimony, to further reassure *Sylvana*.

As already alluded to in some of the examples provided, online contributors also performed solidarity by engaging in affective labor, by displaying emotional availability in their interactions with other people diagnosed with bipolar disorder, and by listening to them with respect and empathy over extended periods of time, judging by the dates and frequency of the comments. At the same time, they showed consideration for the effects their reactions might have upon their interlocutors, or paid attention to the latter's needs and preferences to personalize their advice and render it more appealing. Online contributors also performed solidarity as they sought to motivate people who were going through a difficult time and offered support to those who were experiencing serious mood episodes, as the following exchange illustrates:

> I had already taken the anxiolytics…
>
> But I've managed to ask someone to help me on a forum because I couldn't take it anymore. Someone reacted and we're talking via private messages. I think this will help me a bit. Thanks. (*Derek21*, March 18, 2013)
>
>   *
>
> O.K. If I can also be of any help, it would be my pleasure, even if we haven't talked much…. (*Liane*, March 18, 2013)

The importance of the help online contributors provide each other is highlighted here, as *Derek21* frames the interaction with another person diagnosed with bipolar disorder as an additional therapeutic means to manage anxiety. While *Liane* describes herself as "pathologically pathetic" in her online signature, her reaction suggests that engaging in solidaristic practices online may constitute a way to claim a different identity, that of someone strong and capable enough to support another person with whom she shares an important similarity in a dark moment.

There were, however, also important "costs" to the performance of solidarity. Thus, considerable time was necessary to provide advice and support through well-balanced and carefully considered comments, as was evidenced by replies where contributors acknowledged other people's requests for input, but mentioned that they needed to reflect before providing them with an answer. The provision of information about the effects and side effects of medications that online contributors had taken at some point along their bipolar trajectories required at times rather painful journeys into their past, a revival of periods marked by pain and suffering. Furthermore, people diagnosed with bipolar disorder shared with others with whom they acknowledged certain similarities strategies to manage their condition at the level of daily life, which were often the result of extensive tinkering. While these "costs" were considerable, online contributors underwent them as the insights they put forward not only benefitted others, but also themselves, as they became better aware of their own behaviors and reactions. The identification of important similarities facilitated the development of a new type of collectivity, what I call "digital biocommunities," which I discuss below.

Digital Biocommunities and Their Roles

As the insights provided above illustrated, the online contributors studied here understood their condition in relational terms, by discovering important similarities with others and by making sense of their various experiences through interactions on the fora. The recognition of these commonalities and the performance of solidarity led to an atmosphere of shared intimacy, which made online contributors feel at ease and prompted them to give more detailed and personal information about themselves. This facilitated the development of digital biocommunities, a new type of subgroup that emerged based on increasingly more specific commonalities, including a shared idiom of practice regarding the use of digital technologies. Based on the analysis, it became apparent that the coming into being of this new type of collectivity was underlined by engagements in three types of affective labor: the management of personal affects, the artful display of affective responses, and the careful orchestration of empathy and distance. This way, relations among a growing number of contributors emerged and were maintained and new knowledge could be produced, as people diagnosed with bipolar disorder were able to further their self-knowledge, to perform lay expertise, and to contribute to its collective development.

The attachments and sharing practices developed among the members of these digital biocommunities enabled them to approach their online engagements as reliable ill-health indicators, as the following excerpt illustrates:

> But anyways, I have the feeling that over the last weeks it's been less bad going down [N.B. becoming depressed], so it should be less bad going up [N.B. becoming manic]
> Though when I think about it, I was in such bad shape that I didn't come here anymore…
> It's crazy how much we forget as time goes by…
> What are you up to now? (*Rianne*, February 23, 2015)

Thus, *Rianne* appreciated the severity of her depressive episode by ascribing a considerable weight to her inability to join the forum, as it prompted her to reassess her initial evaluation. For this contributor, participation in this digital biocommunity had become part of how she experienced bipolar disorder, which signals the strength of the social bonds she had developed there.

By developing digital biocommunities, online contributors increasingly related to the digital technologies they used as particular means to act upon disease, as the relative permanence of their posts and the closeness of their interactions with others enabled them to further their self-knowledge and to better manage their condition. This was facilitated by the affordances of fora and by a shared idiom of practice, which allowed for the interpretation of certain online behaviors as markers of particular (ill-health) states. Thus, online contributors could heighten their self-knowledge through their engagements with the posts they had made on the fora over extended periods of time. Since these posts were accompanied by details regarding the time and date when they were made, they functioned as a form of public online diaries, from which people diagnosed with bipolar disorder discerned specific patterns. This allowed them to identify triggers for certain mood episodes, or to improve their assessment of the mood state they experienced, as the following excerpt illustrates:

> it's been the most agonizing thing i've ever experienced. i'd prefer to go through labor and childbirth, because as least when that's over, it's OVER. and besides, it's way less painful than feeling like your soul is being tortured and set on fire.
>
> it will usually begin with a general feeling of anxiety for no discernable reason maybe because i'm bored and don't feel distracted wnough from my evil thoughts. OR something extremely minor will make me IRATE, such as getting curly fries when i asked for regular. by then, it's too late, and i'm angrily yelling and/or throwing my food.
>
> my head starts buzzing with a feeling of electricity/energy, and it feels like a fly is zipping around my brain, bouncing off the inside of my skull. there's an unbearable roar in my brain and i cover my ears, shake my head, and scream/cry. i want to jump out of my skin. i curl up in a ball, in a dark, quiet, small room, and i'm paralyzed there, totally unable to function (…). I want to knock myself unconscious to get rid of the pain, when they are REALLY bad (…)
>
> they are very hard to get out of. and now i'm so manic i'm misspelling evry other word, so i know those aren't even close to all of what is going on inside, but i will surely upset myself if i try to slow down here and think anymore. :-/" (*noone31*, November 6, 2013)

noone31 provides a thick description of her experiences of mixed states by mobilizing highly evocative as well as more broadly relatable comparisons, which help make her state intelligible to others. The last part of her post indicates that elements of online communication, such as misspelling, function for this contributor as markers of a severe manic episode. Furthermore, the way in which the evocative description of her states is organized, its rhythm and punctuation suggest that the post can also be understood as a digital enactment of this mood state. Such practices can therefore be seen as important steps toward achieving self-management and self-change, as they allow disease experiences to be "defined, labeled, and categorized" (Illouz, 2008:196).

Other contributors enhanced their self-knowledge through the substantial knowledge other members of the community had acquired about them, which allowed the latter to mobilize the shared idiom of practice to interpret "deviant" engagements with the technologies of fora as disease markers. For instance, very short replies or the absence of any emoticons across several contributions provided by the same person was seen as a mark of flat affect, and thus indicative of a depressive episode. Similarly, in a context where forum interactions tended to be rather short and to succeed each other quickly, the provision of very long comments, sometimes stretching over the equivalent of six to seven pages, was seen as indicative of a manic episode. The following exchange is illustrative in this sense:

> Vana…are you in good shape or is it just an effect of the screen??? (*Rianne*, March 4, 2015)
>
> *
>
> the optical effect conveys a true reality! I have been in an up [in a manic state] for some time now; I'm even starting to think it's my normal state and nothing will upset it ●(☺)…. (*Sylvana*, March 4, 2015)

The community-building function of the shared idiom of practice comes into relief here through the use of the euphemism "to be in good shape," which for the members of this digital community denoted a manic state, and through the emoticons and brackets at the end of *Sylvana*'s post, which were appropriately interpreted by these contributors. It is important to note the distinct functions fulfilled by the two emoticons and brackets. Through the Red Face emoticon, characteristic for *Doctissimo* (Lombart, 2018), *Sylvana* conveys her anger and exasperation at not being able to manage her feelings, whereas the second emoticon fulfills a relational function, as *Sylvana* uses it to connect with *Rianne*, to express regret about the impact the state she finds herself in may have upon her. This illustrates how affective labor can contribute to the maintenance of one's online network.

Self-knowledge was furthered among the members of digital biocommunities also through the consultations they engaged in, as they actively invited others to help them interpret their experiences and to determine the mood states they were in:

> in favor of the up [manic episode]:
>   I get up every day around 4 pm ◉
>   I started to put on a lot of jewels whereas for months I had only been
> wearing my wedding ring and the one of my deceased mother ◉
>   against the up [manic episode]:
>   I don't feel excited ☺
>   I don't do compulsive shopping ☺
>   I am not aggressive ☺ (*Sylvana,* October 1, 2015)

Sylvana interpellates the other online contributors as experts, who not only have substantial experiential knowledge on bipolar disorder, but also know her very well. She invites them to perform lay expertise by replicating to a certain extent the activities of medical professionals when seeking to establish a diagnosis. Thus, she describes her online and offline behaviors as clues which they can use toward the correct identification of her state. To assist the other online contributors, she places her behaviors in context, providing information about their frequency and about her own emotions in regard to them. Through intensive online interactions with others, *Sylvana* and other contributors like her could bring in relation to bipolar disorder aspects of their behaviors they had not previously considered to be shaped by it, or to identify certain patterns which in time enabled them to better manage this condition. This allowed online contributors to further their self-knowledge, as aspects of the self which may have been opaque or ambiguous to the individual diagnosed with bipolar disorder were clarified relationally. Furthermore, such exchanges may have (had) performative effects on each contributor in ways similar to the narratives disseminated through other media, as signaled by Illouz (2008:185), who argued that one's public illness account "compels him or her to change and to improve his or her condition (…) It makes one responsible for one's future but not for one's past."

In Chap. 4, I have argued that people diagnosed with bipolar disorder could contribute to the development of new insights about the effects and side effects of medications through their online engagements on blogs and fora. The findings described above have cast light upon a different dimension of their contributions, as they indicate that fora can be used to enhance the knowledge online contributors acquire about themselves and others in regard to the manifestations of bipolar disorder and how it shapes their personhood. Such exchanges also enable them to perform lay expertise or to contribute to its collective development, which I will discuss in more detail below.

Solidarity and Lay Expertise

The analysis of the data indicated that lay expertise on bipolar disorder developed as an effect of the solidaristic practices which prompted online contributors to share their embodied, experiential knowledge and the medical insights they had acquired on this condition. The exchange below is a good example in this sense as it illustrates how different contributors came to discover common elements, which moved them to share effective strategies, but also to assume different epistemic positions:

1.Hi everyone, I have bipolar I disorder and

2.have recently experienced being in mixed state the worst I have ever been. It was3.easily the scariest thing I have ever gone through. I was crying uncontrollably at my4.friends house and couldn't stop.

5.I can't explain it to other people very well.

6.My feelings were SO up and down back and forth all at once. The crying wouldn't7.stop.

8.My friends try to be understanding about having bipolar disorder but they struggle to 9.really relate.

10.How can I blame them? I 7.am a bit embarrassed about what happened last week.

11.Does anyone have any tips for me?—Jeanie (*Quickjeanie*, April 5, 2015)

*

1.Hi Quickjeanie, (and welcome), and Gill, I am diagnosed with BP2, rapid cycling, mixed 2.states,

3.and I've definitely experienced those days with the crying jags that accompany an 4.ordinary or slightly hypomanic day.

5.It's defiantly frustrating and confusing.

6.For me its usually something triggers me or I'm under stress when this happens. Or 7.I'm under a medications change or even hormones can do it.

8.I think the best idea for learning about these shifts is to keep a daily journal. You don't 9.have to write full diary entries, but keeping track of your moods, stressors, triggers, 10.medications, even the weather all help you to establish patterns to help you learn to 11.combat these quick shifts. Its also a good tool to take to your Pdoc to be able to 12.discuss these issues with them. I think coping skills you can learn in therapy are a big 13.help as well. Learning some deep breathing exercises, how to identify those triggers, 14.etc. goes a long way to helping the medications.

15.Just know your not alone, and although it's difficult, try not to be to hard on yourself. MO (*midnightowl*, April 5, 2015)

*

1.Jeanie,

2.it sounds like the severity of this particular mixed episode was very unexpected.

3.I believe when something this terrible happens, if we're not at all prepared, it's even 4.worse.

5.How could you prepare for such a thing when you've never had this happen before.

6.I need to make a safety plan for the unexpected episode that could put me in harm's 7.way.

8.Anyone of us could experience what happened to you. Bipolar is unpredictable. Meds 9.and therapy and a host of other wellness skills cannot completely protect us. For me 10.this is why a safety plan is so important.

11.When I have a mixed episode (most all of my bipolar is mixed and also rapid cycle) I 12.don't cry. Pretty much I never cry, even when I want to. My symptoms are extreme 13.agitation and irritability combined with depression.14.There are two things that help: #1. Exercise (this is my first line of defense) #2.

15.Watching a movie (preferably after I've exercised so I'm calm downed enough to enjoy) (*elaine43*, April 5, 2015)

This exchange follows a two-part sequence often encountered in the interactions of psychotherapists with their patients (Wynn & Bergvik, 2010). Thus, a first "troubles-talk" (Jefferson, 1988) sequence, where

Quickjeanie describes her feelings, thoughts, and states to indicate the difficult situation she finds herself in, is followed by a second sequence where *midnightowl* provides a supportive response. Another second sequence is provided, as *elaine43* reacts to *Quickjeanie's* post before the latter has the opportunity to engage with *midnightowl's* statement. While *Quickjeanie* opens her sequence in similar ways to other contributors on the thread, a significant feature of this post is the question at the end, which serves as a direct request for advice based on the same diagnosis and similar experiences. It also indicates that *Quickjeanie* positions herself as a non-expert in regard to the management of this group of symptoms, and considers other forum contributors to be more knowledgeable. By reacting to her post and thereby responding to her interpellation, *midnightowl* and *elaine43* situate themselves as experts in this context, and their posts include various elements meant to justify it. Interesting about the way in which *Quickjeanie* organizes her post is the new theme she introduces in the middle of her description of experienced symptoms (lines 2–4 and 6–7). Through it, this contributor both acknowledges her communicational difficulties and suggests that people who lack experiential knowledge of the symptoms she describes may have a hard time properly understanding them. This is further reinforced by her expectation that people on the forum would be able to provide her with advice others in her immediate surroundings were not able to give her, as denoted by her question.

midnightowl seeks to convey alignment with the experiences recounted by *Quickjeanie* by mirroring to a large extent the organization the latter opted for in her post. Like *Quickjeanie*, she begins her sequence with a greeting, followed by information about her diagnosis, and a description of her experiences with mixed states. This serves both to legitimate her knowledge and to highlight this as an important element she and *Quickjeanie* have in common. This exchange illustrates the careful orchestration of empathy and distance that online contributors engage in to perform lay expertise, as *midnightowl* responds reassuringly to the latter's expectation of empathy (line 5), but moves on to the provision of knowledge, by showing her awareness of particular triggers and by using medical terms. The next and more extensive part of her reply is the response to *Quickjeanie's* direct question, and consists of various suggestions on how the latter could better manage her mixed states. The order of these elements in *midnightowl's* post is important, as the move from personal difficulties to strategies serves to establish her expertise. The authority of her claims thus significantly derives from her ability to successfully, albeit temporarily, address the challenging symptoms she describes and to manage the emotions arising along with them. *midnightowl* concludes her post with a display of solidarity, as she encourages *Quickjeanie* to think of herself as part of a community and provides a caring suggestion in reaction to the latter's statement that she was "a bit embarrassed" by her behavior. The similarity *midnightowl* presumes to exist between her and *Quickjeanie* is further predicated upon common emotions. This is indicated in this part by the preemptive statement "although it's difficult," which signals that *midnightowl* recognizes this affective state, and is aware both of how the contributor might react to this suggestion and of the actual effort required to follow up on it. Such affective labor legitimates the emotions and experiences described by others and lends greater epistemic authority to the advice provided.

elaine43 organizes her reply to *Quickjeanie* in a different way, dedicating a large part of her contribution to the expression of empathy and the display of solidarity. The first sentence is meant to authenticate *Quickjeanie's* experiences as well as to soothe the feelings of embarrassment the latter described. The switch from "I" to "we" in line 3 is important in relation to solidarity, as it shows that *elaine43* thinks of herself, *Quickjeanie*, and presumably other people experiencing difficulties with the management of their symptoms as part of a community, herewith echoing the last part of *midnightowl's* post. At the same time, *elaine43* distinguishes among people diagnosed with bipolar disorder based on their familiarity with the condition, as she pleads to *Quickjeanie* not to feel guilty by framing her as an inexperienced novice. This is a perspective that she nuances by distinguishing between the agency she ascribes people diagnosed with bipolar disorder and the condition itself, as the understanding of bipolar disorder as "unpredictable" and capable of catching off guard any person diagnosed supports her suggestion of creating a safety plan.

This perspective on bipolar disorder contrasts the one advocated by *midnightowl*, who enumerated various options to manage one's condition which she considered effective (lines 8–14), as emphasized through the use of the superlative adjective "best" and of qualifying adjectives with a positive (contextual) value in assessments such as "big help," "good tool," "long way." Without directly interpellating *midnightowl*, *elaine43* engages with the elements in her enumeration, resisting the largely optimistic tone of her message. This move suggests that *elaine43* conceives of solidarity in ways which allow one to have distinct individual experiences while still being part of a large community of sufferers. This can be noted in the positioning of "us" and "for me" next to each other in line 9. It is further reinforced in lines 11–13, where even though the mixed states *elaine43* describes are the opposite of those experienced by *Quickjeanie* and *midnightowl*, she still shares her own coping strategies. This contributor thus seems to base her solidaristic practices on the same diagnosis and to consider this a sufficient commonality for the same strategies to be effective, even when the condition manifests itself differently. Since these elements mirror through their position the location of *Quickjeanie*'s request for advice in her post, they also serve to provide a sense of completion.

In the examples provided above, the performance of lay expertise was achieved through the careful combination of empathy and distance, and the efforts the online contributors were making to manage the flow of affects triggered by the experiences described by others were understated. There were, however, also numerous instances, where the intensity of these affects was in full display, as the following quote illustrates:

> It is true that you are courageous it's amazing I had tears in my eyes [when reading your account].
> I would love to be able to help you but I don't know what to say to you I swear I'm sad for you Vana [N.B.Sylvana]
> I have always said that I didn't want anybody else to know the pains I'm experiencing and now it happens to you and it makes me sad and I feel your pain and I don't know what to do.
> Know that violent noises, fatigue, fear, sadness, anger, anxiety, panic will accentuate your pain. Also the cold as well as burning things. Unlike them, what is soft will relieve your pain...

Don't take too many analgesics because the sleepier you'll feel, the more your muscles will tense. The brain takes it as a signal, like, saying: "Beware! I won't let go of anything!" Have you been advised to take cortisone in low dosages? On my face it works well but on my legs it never led to any results.

Good and sweet night. (*Lera*, April 5, 2015)

This comment thus highlights the affective labor through which the negative affective reactions triggered by *Sylvana's* post—one of the emotional costs of contributing online for people diagnosed with bipolar disorder—are turned into means through which *Lera* can relate to her, while the memory of the latter's own suffering serves to validate *Sylvana's* experiences. Furthermore, *Lera* engages in "caring work," a key form of affective labor (McCosker & Darcy, 2013), to alleviate *Sylvana's* state by expressing empathy, by encouraging and reassuring her. Building upon these affective practices enables her to perform lay expertise, as she advises *Sylvana* on the emotional and physical states that she should avoid to better manage the pain by combining embodied knowledge with medical information.

The personal insights people diagnosed with bipolar disorder shared online and the detailed descriptions of their states and behaviors enabled others to increase their knowledge about this condition in regard to aspects that they did not personally experience, as the quote below illustrates:

How the illness transforms a person....

I know the mixed mood state through you Ria....

I could write volumes about it! I had even strongly thought of it as an outlet it's not bad except that you have to stick to it.

And at the moment concentration is not one of my strengths. (*georgette393*, January 18, 2016)

While no individual diagnosed with bipolar disorder can have experiential knowledge about all the symptoms of this condition, through their frequent interactions with other people diagnosed, online contributors come to develop lay expertise about it and to enrich their personal knowledge through other people's first-hand accounts. This is important, because it shows that these contributors are not only interested in grasping the individual manifestations of their condition, but they want to acquire a thorough understanding of bipolar disorder, which is only possible by accumulating different types of knowledge and by relating their experiences to those of others. Overall, the epistemic relevance of these insights was often publicly acknowledged, as the following excerpt illustrates:

> Thank you for your personal experiences you have helped me understand a lot more about myself. I only wish my clinical psych was as clear about this as the information I've managed to understand here. (*Polar1, May 18,* 2016)

Discussion

This chapter has shown that despite individualizing tendencies in personalized and precision medicine, solidarity remains an important value for people diagnosed with bipolar disorder and it underlies the performance and collective development of lay expertise. Thus, rather than focusing on the distinctions between themselves and others, the online contributors studied here identified important similarities with each other, which prompted them to incur personal costs in order to provide others with help and support. To account for this innovative coming together, I put forward the concept of digital biocommunities to denote the development of (sub)groups based on numerous commonalities of experience and similar engagements with the technologies of fora. By developing digital biocommunities, online contributors related to the digital technologies they used as particular means to act upon disease. While such statements are nowadays often made in relation to digital mental health applications, which provide quantified insights or visualizations, this chapter has illustrated that people's ability to manage bipolar disorder is enhanced through the narratives, thick descriptions, and dialogue that fora and similar interactive online platforms allow for. Online contributors can further their self-control and better navigate daily life through the practices of self-revelation/clarification and collective consultation in which they engage. In so doing, they also contribute to the development of lay expertise about this condition, as a more unified and comprehensive image of bipolar disorder and its manifestations at the personal level emerges through frequent online exchanges.

The development of lay expertise traced here depended not only on epistemic practices, but also on the ability of online contributors to appeal to the considerations, emotions, and perspectives of their interlocutors, and on their display of sympathy and empathy. The sharing of experiential and other types of knowledge required for the development of lay expertise was also informed by the feelings of well-being that online contributors experienced in so doing, as they could temporarily position themselves as knowledgeable, capable, and supportive rather than frail, vulnerable, and in need of help. Thus, for knowledge to be shared, circulated, and produced, it was not enough for people diagnosed to identify relevant similarities, but they also needed to engage in the affective labor required when interacting publicly with multiple individuals. Affective practices and engagements play therefore an important role in the production of knowledge, even though these aspects have been thus far largely neglected in social studies of science. Furthermore, the findings discussed here illustrated that affective labor is more than unpaid work, as, through it, online contributors could perform a value they found important; they acquired self-knowledge and contributed to the development of collective knowledge on the management of bipolar disorder.

The close link between solidarity and lay expertise that these findings illustrated is important in the current context where knowledge is increasingly referred to as a resource that can be privately owned (Newell, 2015) and is thus more often related to other values, such as competitiveness and efficiency. Nevertheless, it is important to bear in mind that solidarity is not in itself a positive value (Dean, 1995). As people come together with others with whom they share important similarities and are willing to incur costs in order to assist them, they also distinguish themselves from those with whom they do not share such similarities. Such tendencies could also be noted in this chapter, as some online contributors distinguished in essential ways between people who were diagnosed with bipolar disorder and those who were not. While such processes of inclusion and exclusion may not be prevented, for digital biocommunities to continue to have positive effects, it is important that their members reflect upon the criteria they use to include and exclude others and upon the consequences such practices may have.

Digital biocommunities bear some resemblance to self-help groups, which in the past have facilitated the development of a common identity among people diagnosed with contested conditions, such as the fibromyalgia syndrome (Barker, 2002). This is in line with previous findings that have shown that online communities share with their offline predecessors similar objectives, work practices, modes of approach, and orientation toward cognitive resources (Akrich, 2010). The development of digital biocommunities can be interpreted as indicative of a growing need among people diagnosed to come together, share experiences, and support each other in a context marked by the increased deregularization of mental healthcare services. This is supported by the fact that both in the US and in France the number of self-help and support groups, described in more detail in Chap. 2, has been increasing over the last few decades (Fox, 2011; Girard, 2008). Since background conditions can further or deter solidaristic practices (Prainsack & Buyx, 2017), more research is needed to understand how they affect online engagements, and what role the different affordances and designs of fora and other interactive online platforms play in such developments and what types of solidarity are thereby encouraged.

While self-help groups have been historically less influential in France than in the US, solidarity is considered by many to be a national value in France, which might explain the more numerous and frequent exchanges to support others in need on the *Troubles Bipolaires* threads. The role of cultural and social factors in explaining such distinct online behaviors was further reinforced by the fact that on two other American fora, which were consulted to compare the number of participants and their interactions, few threads exceeded 30 comments, let alone reach hundreds or thousands. The distinct online landscape available for both countries may have been another influencing element, as infrastructural, economic, and institutional factors have shaped the development of a dispersed online environment in the US and a more centralized one in France. Future studies are therefore needed to acquire a better understanding of the specific factors that inform such differences in online participation and support between contributors from the US and France.

The solidaristic practices described in this chapter were identified at a time when the pronounced individualization of responsibility brought about by personalized and precision medicine has led many scholars to approach solidarity as a value that is under threat and in need of protection (Aarden et al., 2010). The resilience of solidarity in this context indicates that it is a very important value to people, who find solace in knowing that they are not alone in experiencing specific issues. The concept of digital biocommunities suggests that as people come together based on increasingly more specific commonalities of experience, they might form part of multiple dynamic (sub)groups, depending on the similarities they focus upon and the solidaristic practices they engage in. This has consequences for the ways in which personhood and "personalization" are understood, as it strengthens the idea that they are defined and re-defined through social interactions and practices which are meaningful to people diagnosed. Hopefully, through their multitude and diversity, the development of digital biocommunities will provide people diagnosed with bipolar disorder with safe havens, where they can feel at ease and where they can become better aware of their talents, strengths, and knowledge, and of the important values they uphold as they share them with others.

References

Aarden, E., van Hoyweghen, I., & Horstman, K. (2010). Solidarity in Practices of Provision: Distributing Access to Genetic Technologies in Health Care in Germany, the Netherlands and the United Kingdom. *New Genetics and Society, 29*(4), 369–388.

Akrich, M. (2010). From Communities of Practice to Epistemic Communities: Health Mobilizations on the Internet. *Sociological Research Online, 15*(2), 10. Available at http://www.socresonline.org.uk/15/2/10.html

Akrich, M., Méadel, C., & Rémy, C. (2008). Building Collectives via the Web? Information and Mobilization on Cancer Websites. *Virtually Informed, 2008*, 13–40.

Andersson, Y. (2017). Blogs and the Art of Dying: Blogging With, and About, Severe Cancer in Late Modern Swedish Society. *OMEGA-Journal of Death and Dying, 79*, 1–20. https://doi.org/10.1177/0030222817719806

Armstrong, N., Koteyko, N., & Powell, J. (2012). "Oh Dear, Should I Really Be Saying That on Here?" Issues of Identity and Authority in an Online Diabetes Community. *Health, 16*(4), 347–365.

Barker, K. (2002). Self-Help Literature and the Making of an Illness Identity: The Case of Fibromyalgia Syndrome (FMS). *Social Problems, 49*(3), 279–300.

Bayertz, K. (Ed.). (1998). *Solidarität: Begriff und Problem*. Suhrkamp.

Baylis, F., Kenny, N., & Sherwin, S. (2008). A Relational Account of Public Health Care Ethics. *Public Health Ethics, 1*(3), 196–209.

Clough, P. (2008). The Affective Turn. Political Economy, Biomedia and Bodies. *Theory, Culture & Society, 25*(1), 1–22.

Dean, J. (1995). Reflective Solidarity. *Constellations, 2*(1), 114–140.

Dickenson, D. (2013). *Me Medicine vs. We Medicine: Reclaiming Biotechnology for the Common Good*. Columbia University Press.

Durkheim, E. (1964). *The Division of Labor in Society*. Free Press.

Epstein, S. (2007). *Inclusion. The Politics of Difference in Medical Research*. The University of Chicago Press.

Etzioni, A. (1988). *The Moral Dimension. Toward a New Economics*. Free Press.

Evers, K. (2009). Personalized Medicine in Psychiatry: Ethical Challenges and Opportunities. *Dialogues in Clinical Neuroscience, 11*(4), 427–434.

Foster, C. (2009). *Choosing Life, Choosing Death: The Tyranny of Autonomy in Medical Ethics and Law*. Hart.

Fox, S. (2011). *Peer-to-peer healthcare*. California Healthcare.

Gershon, I. (2010). *The Breakup 2.0. Disconnecting over New Media*. Cornell University Press. E-book.

Girard, V. (2008). Dossier n° 13- Auto Support en Santé Mentale en France. *Bulletin Amades, 75*, 1–9.

Hardt, M. (1999). Affective Labor. *Boundary, 26*(2), 89–100.

Hardt, M., & Negri, A. (2004). *Multitude. War and Democracy in the Age of Empire*. The Penguin Press.

Hechter, M. (1987). Nationalism as Group Solidarity. *Ethnic and Racial Studies, 10*(4), 415–426.

Hedgecoe, A. (2004). *The Politics of Personalised Medicine: Pharmacogenetics in the Clinic*. Cambridge University Press.

Hochschild, A. (2012). *The Managed Heart. Commercialization of Human Feeling* (3rd ed.). University of California Press.

Hogle, L. (2016). Data-intensive Resourcing in Healthcare. *BioSocieties, 11*(3), 372–393.

Illouz, E. (2008). *Saving the Modern Soul. Therapy, Emotions, and the Culture of Self-Help*. University of California Press.

Illouz, E. (2018). *Emotions as Commodities. Capitalism, Consumption and Authenticity*. Routledge.

Kaufman, S., & Whitehead, K. (2016). Producing, Ratifying, and Resisting Support in an Online Support Forum. *Health*, 1–17. Advance online publication. https://doi.org/10.1177/1363459315628043

Kitzman, A. (2004). *Saved from Oblivion: Documenting the Daily from Diaries to Web Cams*. Peter Lang.

Kneese, T. (2017). Mediating Mortality: Transtemporal Illness Blogs and Digital Care Work. In S. Boret, S. Long, & S. Kan (Eds.), *Death in the Early Twenty-First Century* (pp. 179–213). Palgrave Macmillan.

Knoppers, B., & Chadwick, R. (2005). Human Genetic Research: Emerging Trends in Ethics. *Nature, 6*, 75–79.

Komter, A. (2005). *Social Solidarity and the Gift*. Cambridge University Press.

Lombart, E. (2018). The Emoticon Functions in Antiphrasis Interpretation on Doctissimo's Forums. In L.-A. Cougnon, B. De Cock, & C. Fairon (Eds.), *Language and the New (instant) Media* (pp. 1–17). Presses Universitaires de Louvain.

Lupton, D. (2014). The Commodification of Patient Opinion: The Digital Patient Experience Economy in the Age of Big Data. *Sociology of Health & Illness, 36*(6), 856–869.

Lupton, D. (2016). *The Quantified Self. A Sociology of Self-Tracking*. Polity Press.

Lupton, D. (2018). *Digital Health*. Routledge.

Lussier, K. (2018). Temperamental Workers: Psychology, Business, and the Humm-Wadsworth Temperament Scale in Interwar America. *History of Psychology, 21*(2), 79–99.

Mayhew, L. (1971). *Society: Institutions and Activity*. Columbia University Press.

McCosker, A. (2018). Engaging Mental Health Online: Insights from *beyondblue*'s forum influencers. *New Media & Society, 20*(12), 4748–4764.

McCosker, A., & Darcy, R. (2013). Living with Cancer. Affective Labour, Self-Expression and the Utility of Blogs. *Information, Communication & Society, 16*(8), 1266–1285.

Mitchell, R., & Waldby, C. (2010). National Biobanks: Clinical Labor, Risk Production, and the Creation of Biovalue. *Science, Technology & Human Values, 35*(3), 330–355.

Newell, S. (2015). Managing Knowledge and Managing Knowledge Work: What We Know and What the Future Holds. *Journal of Information Technology, 30*, 1–17.

Nussbaum, M. (2003). *Upheavals of Thought: The Intelligence of Emotions*. Cambridge University Press.

Ozomaro, U., Wahlestedt, C., & Nemeroff, C. (2013). Personalized Medicine in Psychiatry: Problems and Promises. *BMC Medicine, 11*, 132.

Parsons, T. (1952). *The Social System.* Tavistock.

Prainsack, B. (2017). *Personalized Medicine. Empowered Patients in the 21ˢᵗ Century?* New York University Press.

Prainsack, B., & Buyx, A. (2012). Solidarity in Contemporary Bioethics — Towards a New Approach. *Bioethics, 26*(7), 343–350.

Prainsack, B., & Buyx, A. (2017). *Solidarity in Biomedicine and Beyond.* Cambridge University Press.

Rabeharisoa, V., & Callon, M. (2002). The Involvement of Patients' Associations in Research. *ISSJ, 171*, 57–65.

Rabeharisoa, V., Moreira, T., & Akrich, M. (2013). Evidence-based Activism: Patients' Organizations, Users' and Activist's Groups in Knowledge Society. *CSI Working Papers Series, 033*, 1–27.

Rabinow, P. (1996). *Essays on the Anthropology of Reason.* Princeton University Press.

Sharon, T. (2017). Self-tracking for Health and the Quantified Self: Re-articulating Autonomy, Solidarity and Authenticity in an Age of Personalized Healthcare. *Philosophy & Technology, 30*(1), 93–121.

Shin, C., Han, C., Pae, C., & Patkar, A. (2016). Precision Medicine for Psychopharmacology: A General Introduction. *Expert Review of Neurotherapeutics, 16*(7), 831–839.

Sosnowy, C. (2014). Practicing Patienthood Online: Social Media, Chronic Illness, and Lay Expertise. *Societies, 4*, 316–329.

Steinhubl, S., Muse, E., & Topol, E. (2013). Can Mobile Health Technologies Transform Health Care? *JAMA, 310*(22), 2395–2396.

Swan, M. (2009). Emerging Patient-Driven Health Care Models: An Examination of Health Social Networks, Consumer Personalized Medicine and Quantified Self-Tracking. *International Journal of Environmental Research and Public Health, 6*(2), 492–525.

Swierstra, T. (2013). Nanotechnology and Techno-Moral Change. *Ethics & Politics, 15*(1), 200–219.

Terranova, T. (2000). Free Labor: Producing Culture for the Digital Economy. *Social Text 63, 18*(2), 33–58.

Topol, E. (2015). *The Patient Will See You Now. The Future of Medicine Is in Your Hands.* Basic Books.

Van de Werff, T. (2018). *Practicing the Plastic Brain. Popular Neuroscience and the Good Life.* Datawyse.

Van Dijck, J. (2013). *The Culture of Connectivity. A Critical History of Social Media*. Oxford University Press.

Van Hoyweghen, I., & Rebert, L. (2012). Your Genes in Insurance: From Generic Discrimination to Genomic Solidarity. *Personalized Medicine, 9*(8), 871–877.

Van Oorschot, W., & Komter, A. (1998). What Is That Ties...? Theoretical Perspectives on Social Bond. *Sociale Wetenschappen, 41*(3), 4–24.

Waldby, C., & Cooper, M. (2008). The Biopolitics of Reproduction. *Australian Feminist Studies, 23*(55), 57–73.

Weber, M. (1947). *The Theory of Social and Economic Organization*. Free Press. Translated by A.M. Henderson & Talcott Parsons.

Weber, G., Mandl, K., & Kohane, I. (2014). Finding the Missing Link for Big Biomedical Data. *JAMA, 311*(24), 2479–2480.

Wium-Anderesen, I., Vinberg, M., Kessing, L., & McIntyre, R. (2017). Personalized Medicine in Psychiatry. *Nordic Journal of Psychiatry, 71*(1), 12–19.

Wynn, R., & Bergvik, S. (2010). Studying Empathy as an Interactional Three-Part Sequence. *Patient Education and Counseling, 80*(1), 150.

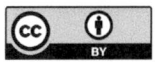

7

Expertise in the Age of Big Data

The study described in this book was motivated by important debates about the meaning and the effects of major transformations that expertise has undergone in Western societies. Over the last few decades, expertise has come to occupy a rather paradoxical position. On the one hand, we are surrounded by *more* expertise because ever more domains of our lives have come under the authority of "experts" and because expertise has been increasingly claimed by "non-experts," by people lacking official accreditations. On the other hand, the right and authority of experts to make decisions that impact the lives of many and the grounds upon which such decisions are made have been called into question, as the rise in anti-elitist and populist feelings over the last decade indicates. We live, therefore, at a time, when expertise is both ubiquitous and very much challenged. The Internet has played an important role in these developments, as it has provided new avenues for the production, dissemination, and evaluation of knowledge. Since this medium has been widely used by a broad range of stakeholders in the field of mental health, throughout this book I have scrutinized the different ways in which it has shaped the performance of expertise about bipolar disorder.

The use of the Internet in mental healthcare has given rise to numerous fears and expectations. Some have hailed this medium's potential to help

© The Author(s) 2023
C. Egher, *Digital Healthcare and Expertise*, Health, Technology and Society,
https://doi.org/10.1007/978-981-16-9178-2_7

improve the accessibility and affordability of mental health therapies and have also welcomed the possibility it affords people diagnosed to come together and exchange insights with others with the same diagnosis. Others have worried about the varying quality of online mental health-related information and about the ways in which such insights may affect relations between medical professionals and people diagnosed, which have been rather strained historically. These fears and hopes are to a certain extent well founded, yet they neglect the multiple, dynamic character the Internet can have as well as the different forms of engagement users can take up online, depending on their personal interests, skills, and goals, as well as on the social and cultural perspectives which shape their understanding of specific mental health conditions. In this book, I have tried to reconcile the agency of users with a perspective which sees online technologies as value-laden and capable of actively influencing people's behaviors. This way I have been able to compare the ways in which different stakeholders seek to make their expertise manifest by using different online technologies and I have scrutinized how the design and online affordances available on different online platforms shape such performances. I have also investigated the transformations that such online engagements may lead to in the relations between people diagnosed and medical professionals, and have probed the individualizing or collectivity-generating effects the Internet can have in regard to the online performance of expertise. Furthermore, I have also focused on how different cultural norms and values inform these transformations.

The main finding of this book is that the online performance of expertise is not a straightforward process by which offline practices, tools, and approaches are transferred online, but involves additional skills and complex negotiations, which sometimes lead to unexpected configurations. Despite expectations that the availability of health-related information would lead to patient empowerment and would allow people diagnosed to re-position themselves in relation to medical professionals, the findings presented here have revealed a more complex picture, where individuals diagnosed with bipolar disorder can become highly influential through their skillful use of the Internet and by developing and cultivating important alliances with "traditional" experts. Contrary to expectations that the focus on "radical" differences in personalized and precision medicine would lead to increased individualization, online contributors diagnosed with bipolar disorder performed solidarity with others with whom they shared numerous similarities, which prompted them to engage in epistemic practices as well as affective labor. These findings prompted the development of a new conceptualization of expertise, understood as a practical and collective achievement, realized through coordination and affective labor among stakeholders who occupy multiple and shifting positions within a complex ecosystem.

Each of the empirical chapters has highlighted different ways in which expertise on bipolar disorder was performed online by various stakeholders. In this chapter, these findings are brought together and reflected upon to consider what they can tell us about the meaning and relevance of expertise in the context where promises generated by big data analytics suggest that substantial knowledge no longer describes (solely) a set of human capabilities and may no longer require human intervention in order to be applied in a variety of contexts. I highlight what the findings presented in the empirical chapters mean in relation to the key questions this book has addressed.

The Online Performance of Expertise About Bipolar Disorder

Different Stakeholder's Use of the Internet

One of the unambiguous conclusions of this study is that different stakeholders used online technologies differently and that the choice thereof was not only informed by the resources at their disposal, but also by their goals and priorities. Thus, the analysis revealed that even though the National Institute of Mental Health (NIMH) and La Haute Autorité de Santé (HAS), the two governmental institutions studied in this book, have vast financial and technical resources at their disposal, they are reluctant Internet users, who have opted for non-interactive platforms and for conservative online technologies. I have argued that such an approach allowed them to push perspectives and research orientations that were no longer popular to the background, and it also enabled them to obscure from view the disagreements and struggles between different medical professionals who study or provide medical care for this condition. Furthermore, the choice for non-interactive platforms made it possible for them to share their perspectives about bipolar disorder authoritatively and without directly addressing the challenges brought to psychiatry by people diagnosed, their families, and even medical professionals. These governmental agencies used, however, different online tools, which were better aligned with their main goals and audiences. For instance, through the affordances available on the pdf files HAS provided, such as the audio option and the ruler, I have argued that this governmental agency used its platform for very specific educational purposes, meant to facilitate information retention and decision-making in clinical practice. The insights acquired from the empirical analyses discussed in the other chapters of this book suggest, however, that these governmental agencies need to consider the heterogeneity of the population they address in their online performance of expertise about bipolar disorder. While no access could be secured to find out how the information posted online was developed and by whom, studying how aspects of the identity of those designing and implementing this information shape their work and affect the envisaged users would be a fruitful direction for future research.

Unlike the governmental agencies discussed, people diagnosed with bipolar disorder used blogs and fora, where they could share their doubts and insights, either by initiating forum threads or by commenting on blog posts or threads written by others. It was shown that this allows for a bottom-up accumulation of perspectives and for a dialogical performance of expertise, as various treatment experiences, the advantages and disadvantages of various therapeutic approaches, and the results of self-experiments can be extensively discussed among numerous contributors. Whereas the people diagnosed studied in Chap. 4 used the Internet to share their treatment experiences and to acquire specific information, the online contributors studied in Chap. 6 used fora to come together and support others with whom they shared important commonalities. I have shown that how they engaged with the affordances available on these online platforms played an important role in the development of digital biocommunities, as it constituted a relevant similarity and reinforced sharing practices among the members of such groups. This way members of such communities came to use these online platforms as public diaries, through which they and their readers could keep track of developments in their mental, physical, and emotional states.

The different reasons people diagnosed with bipolar disorder chose to use the Internet also led to different dynamics. In general, online contributors interested in specific information shared their treatment experiences across one or several exchanges within a brief period of time and returned sometimes after a long interval to share new insights. In contrast, people interested in developing closer ties with others put a lot of time and effort into sharing their experiences online and reacting to those of others, either on the main page of the fora and/or through private messages with specific contributors. Only a very limited number of medical professionals have shared their insights on the platforms studied here, which has prevented the development of clear perspectives on how they use the Internet to acquire or share information about bipolar disorder. Since the prevalence of this condition suggests that a considerable number of medical professionals must also be diagnosed with bipolar disorder, it would be relevant to find out more about their perspectives in this regard and on the ways in which they call upon their different types of knowledge to perform expertise about bipolar disorder online. Even though the concept of performance implies that meaning comes into being through the efforts of the actors and of the audience, through the interactions between users and the various elements of online interfaces (Drucker, 2010), it was not possible to conduct interviews or to observe users within the same physical space. Addressing this aspect in future studies would lead to important contributions.

People Diagnosed, Medical Professionals, and the Internet

The findings discussed in this book also indicated that the Internet is not a neutral medium through which expertise about bipolar disorder can be performed, but that it shapes in some notable ways the position people diagnosed can occupy in relation to medical professionals. Through the use of blogs and fora, people diagnosed with bipolar disorder were able to engage in processes of knowledge production about this condition, thereby acquiring more influence and agency. As discussed in Chap. 4, through their online affordances which allow for the longitudinal accumulation in the same spaces of numerous insights, blogs and fora facilitated the development of what I have called "digitally informed hypotheses" about the effects and side effects of medications. This may have immediate empowering effects for individual users, by confirming the importance of their insights and thereby encouraging them to assume a more confident position in their interactions with medical professionals. In other cases, online platforms seemed to represent therapeutic approaches in themselves, as getting in touch with other people diagnosed and talking to them about their issues was often framed as contributing to one's well-being and mental stability. Also from this point of view, the Internet appeared to empower some online contributors, as it assisted them in developing more agency over bipolar disorder. If recognized by relevant others, such as family members, medical professionals, and current or potential employers, this ability of people diagnosed to better manage their condition could, in turn, improve their quality of life by leading to more equal relations and more collaborative exchanges.

As people with different understandings of bipolar disorder, who had different relations with their medical professionals and different needs and possibilities in their daily life, came together online, even in brief exchanges, the Internet may also have contributed toward a more open dialogue about this condition. In time, this may lead to the development of new standards to determine what accounts for reliable information at a more general level. Importantly, while at the moment the "digitally informed hypotheses" described in Chap. 4 require the assistance of medical professionals to become clinical evidence, in time this may no longer be necessary. As the integration of different types of data fueled by personalized and precision medicine may develop further, the insights provided by people diagnosed through their online interactions may come to be recognized as clinical evidence, even in the absence of significant interventions from medical professionals. Should this occur, it will be difficult to deny the contribution of blogs and fora in enabling people diagnosed with bipolar disorder to re-position themselves more authoritatively in relation to medical professionals, as these platforms facilitated the production of new knowledge and will have thus shaped the prescription of treatment for this condition.

Nevertheless, Chap. 5 showed that while the Internet does not always favor the powerful, only a small number of individuals are able to re-position themselves and to acquire a high standing. The two bloggers studied in this chapter managed through the skillful use of this medium to become highly influential. Through their popularity, visibility, and credibility, Tracy and Fast not only shape how their readers understand and approach bipolar disorder, but also influence the production of knowledge about this condition, as they engage in productive collaborations with medical professionals. Yet, these bloggers did not use their standing to further democratize participation in the production of knowledge. Rather than promoting research projects developed by citizen scientists or various crowdsourced initiatives, Tracy and Fast informed their readers about projects undertaken by medical professionals with whom they were familiar, or with whom they personally collaborated. Through the efforts they made to familiarize readers with scientific methodology and through their advice on how to best approach medical professionals, these bloggers may, nonetheless, have already helped their readers develop more collaborative relations with the latter and may have facilitated the participation of a greater number of people diagnosed with bipolar disorder in research.

The data used in the study described in this book were collected from blog posts and forum threads with many comments; thus, the insights provided on the selected online platforms may be more representative of people's experiences with certain therapeutic approaches than others. Focusing on the content made available on online platforms with limited (public) interactions and comparing differences in online interactivity in relation to various forms of treatment would therefore be a promising avenue for future research. Furthermore, since the results presented here are based on the experiences of readers who were motivated enough to contribute online, they do not represent all people diagnosed with bipolar disorder. More studies are therefore needed to understand the perspectives of people who use interactive online platforms for information purposes but refrain from contributing and those of people who refuse to use the Internet for health-related purposes or who do not have access to it. Studying the impact online contributions have on readers and how lasting their effects are among other online participants would also provide valuable contributions to the literature. To better understand how people diagnosed with bipolar disorder re-position themselves in relation to medical professionals through their use of the Internet, offline ethnographic studies on how medical professionals make sense of such online engagements, how online expertise is brought to medical settings, and the consequences this has are needed.

Cultural Markers and Expertise on Bipolar Disorder Online

The findings presented in this book suggest that local norms and values play an important role in how expertise on bipolar disorder is performed online. Content-wise, the differences between the contributions on American and French online platforms were largely shaped by the ways in which mental healthcare was organized in these countries and by the preferred scientific approach to bipolar disorder. Thus, differences in the insurance system lead to different uses and engagements with the technologies of online platforms. For (temporarily) uninsured American contributors, online platforms constituted valuable alternatives or stand-ins for medical professionals, as these contributors relied upon the advice of other people diagnosed to identify affordable and effective medications and to determine some alternative practices they could take up, to heighten their chances to remain stable. Furthermore, discussions about generic drugs and their different effects were very popular on American blogs and fora, but did not occupy a prominent position on French platforms. In contrast, many French contributors worried about overmedication in France, as surveys positioned France among the countries with the highest consumption rates in Europe. Another noteworthy difference concerns the social impact ascribed to bipolar disorder. Whereas most American contributors framed this condition as a disability which prevented them from gaining or maintaining meaningful employment, many French contributors were employed, at times in highly demanding positions.

The relations between medical professionals and people diagnosed seemed fairly balanced on French platforms, with some contributors confessing to more strained relations and denouncing the practice of forced hospitalization, while many others expressed trust in their medical professionals and described their interactions with them as collaborations, even though between unequal partners. In contrast, on American platforms there were more pronounced tendencies for people diagnosed to complain about the quality of medical care they received, to highlight the lack of trust medical professionals displayed toward their experiences with medications. While some contributors explained such strained relations by invoking the close financial links between psychiatrists and pharmaceutical companies, there were also many who ascribed them to the different levels of expertise of different medical professionals. Furthermore, in the US, the antipsychiatry movement seemed to have remained influential enough to be taken up on many of the blogs and fora studied. In France, psychoanalysis was still considered a possible therapeutic approach, making its presence felt through the use of its terminology in discussions about the causes of bipolar disorder and about the elements that may affect people's response to treatment.

There were also important differences regarding the preferred types of online technologies people diagnosed with bipolar disorder from these countries used. Whereas in the US, blogs acquired more readers and more comments, in France, fora were by far the most popular, with an impressive number of readers and online contributions. There was also a notable difference regarding the extent to which online and offline practices were integrated in the US and France. In contrast to French contributors, most American online contributors rarely used blogs and fora to organize offline events or to inform readers about them. More studies are needed to acquire a better understanding of the factors that account for such differences in the use of online platforms and their affordances among American and French online contributors, and of the standing the latter may come to occupy online.

The Internet and its Individualizing or Collectivity-Generating Effects in Relation to Expertise

This book has shown that the Internet has both individualizing and collectivity-generating effects in relation to expertise, as people diagnosed with bipolar disorder shared their insights on this condition online. The analysis in Chap. 4 showed that the Internet can contribute to the development of new individual-group configurations. The online contributors studied shared their treatment experiences as individuals rather than representatives of certain groups, and their interactions with others were most of the time too fleeting for actual communities to develop. Nevertheless "light" forms of collectives did come into being. Such collectives did not develop, however, through the agency of the online contributors alone, but were facilitated by the online affordances of blogs and fora, which allowed for the accumulation of their insights in the same spaces. Importantly, even though online contributors could decide never to return to a specific online platform again, unless they deleted their contribution, they continued to be part of that collective long after their last visit, through the insights they had shared. Furthermore, certain online affordances available on these platforms may further serve as reminders of their participation, as notifications about new comments or about specific reactions to their own contributions may allow people diagnosed to keep track of reactions on that platform, even when they no longer participate actively.

Closely knit collectives could also develop online, as was shown in Chap. 6. I have termed such (sub)groups "digital biocommunities" to highlight the fact that they are not only brought together by increasingly more specific commonalities of experience, but also by shared approaches to the digital technologies used. Thus, online contributors were drawn together by similar interests, as they reacted to specific forum threads, by common attitudes about their condition and the social-political circumstances they were living in, which they could refer to in brief or more elaborate forms through the use of specific online affordances available on these platforms. In contrast, Chap. 5 revealed that the use of the

Internet contributes to the development of a new type of individual stakeholder, what I have called "online expert mediators." This new stakeholder category emerges at the intersection between the diagnosis of bipolar disorder, the acquisition of particular types of knowledge, and an individual's skillful use of the Internet. It has also been made possible by the limited trust some of the people diagnosed and their families have toward medical professionals due to various scandals over the last two decades regarding the close ties between psychiatrists and pharmaceutical companies. The rise of online expert mediators may mark a turn from community activism to exceptional entrepreneurial selves. This book has therefore described a new form of individualization as well as a new form of collectivization that the Internet contributed to, and has shown that both forms exist simultaneously online.

By using the concept of interactional expertise to study the activities of these online expert mediators, expertise about bipolar disorder was approached as the property of individuals. In so doing, however, the role of medical professionals and other people from whom these bloggers learned before starting their own blog and the inspiration and new insights they acquired from the contributors on their platforms were not taken into account. While it may well be that Fast is right and that readers "appreciate quality above all else" (e-mail interview, 2016), more studies on the behavior of different online audiences and their online preferences are needed, to understand what such popularity is based on. Given that socioeconomic inequalities have been shown to influence the quality of (professional) care one receives when healthcare is provided through public–private partnerships (Engel & Van Lente, 2014), it is necessary to understand whether online expert mediators represent a cheap(er) way to access medical information for people with limited resources or an additional means through which those sufficiently well-off may seek to manage their health. As the concerns discussed in Chap. 2 in regard to digital and AI-based technologies highlighted, the Internet could also contribute to harming online contributors on "free" platforms, if the platform owners sell such data to employers, insurance companies, banks, and other institutions that importantly shape one's quality of life.

Knowledge Production in the Digital Age: Contributions

In this section, the significance of the findings described above is discussed by considering their relevance in regard to processes of knowledge production in the digital age and to the role the Internet plays in them. In so doing, I argue that we need to move beyond rather simplistic approaches which see the Internet either as a quick technological fix or as a postmodern version of Pandora's box.

The findings presented in this book are the result of a qualitative study, which focused on the narrative accounts provided by various stakeholders on different types of online platforms. Yet, as was highlighted in Chap. 2, this research unfolded against a background where developments in digital technologies and data analytics have led many to believe that the days of the relevance of human knowledge as we know it are counted. As we have seen, enthusiastic about the capacities and potential of high-performing intelligent machines, such commentators—often developers or owners of digital companies—believe the acquisition of huge amounts of data from numerous individuals (will) enable computers and algorithms to provide better, more relevant solutions to all sorts of problems (Mayer-Schönberger & Cukier, 2013). Such processes are underlined by a shift from causation to correlation in the development of knowledge, as such technologies can process at great speed previously unimaginable volumes of data, and identify relevant patterns. The insights thus acquired are appealing to many, especially to those who find themselves at sufficient distance from these technologies, not only because of the remarkable calculations upon which they are based, but also because of their apparent objectivity, as human bias is (mistakenly) thought to be largely removed from them. Such digital technologies are thought to become better alternatives to human expertise because of the many flaws that are imputed to human professionals, such as their insufficient or fragmented access to information, their limited capacities to process all relevant data and to make accurate predictions about complex phenomena, and their difficulty to overcome personal or collective ideologies and interests (Topol, 2019). In this context, knowledge produced by digital technologies and algorithms is made to shine brighter, due to its perceived neutrality and objectivity.

This book told, however, a different story, as it emphasized the importance of several typically human competencies, such as sensitivity to context, norms, and values, for the performance of expertise. By studying how governmental agencies and people diagnosed with bipolar disorder performed expertise online, I argued that expertise could better be approached as a practical achievement, realized through coordination and affective labor among stakeholders with different types of knowledge, who occupy multiple shifting positions across a complex ecosystem. One of the merits of this conceptualization is that it focuses on affective labor, showing that it plays an important role in epistemic practices. This is particularly important in the current context, where big data enthusiasts have started to invoke affective practices to argue in favor of using artificial intelligence (AI) in medical practice. Thus, Topol (2019) claims that the use of AI as diagnostic tools would free up time for medical professionals to be more "present," "humane," and "empathetic" during their encounters with patients. Furthermore, he argues that "it is essential that we upgrade diagnosis from an art to a digital-driven science" (Topol, 2019: Loc. 893). As this last statement shows, such visions do not consider affective labor and practices as part of (medical) expertise, of epistemic practices, but rather as something different, that can be separated from the former, and that can be called upon and managed.

The findings presented in this book have shown, however, that affective labor is closely tied to the development and performance of expertise and that this relation is not limited to people diagnosed (Chap. 6) but also mobilized in the development and translation of knowledge among different communities of practice (Chap. 5). Thus, affective practices, creativity, and adaptability are typically human capabilities that have been shown to play a significant role in the production of knowledge, as well as in its accurate interpretation and successful implementation. This is in line with arguments developed by Collins (2018) in his study on artificial intelligence, where he highlights the importance of context sensitivity and language acquisition in regard to expertise. In his opinion, such abilities can only be acquired through acculturation in a given society and are importantly tied, from a collective point of view, to embodiment, to the ways in which one makes sense of the world with and through one's body. Furthermore, Collins emphasizes that in their interactions with others, people constantly engage in substantial, highly complex forms of "repair work," as they make sense of, adapt, fill in, and modify the broken and incomplete information they receive, in order to develop appropriate responses. The findings presented in Chap. 4 of this book support this perspective, because they highlighted the adaptative character of expertise, as general views on the effectiveness of medications or on the manifestations of bipolar disorder were enriched by being assessed and applied to the specific circumstances, needs, and preferences of various individuals. That epistemic practices are also affective in various ways is important not only from a scientific point of view, but also politically, especially given the skewed gendered distribution and income inequality characterizing professions where care rather than knowledge is highlighted (Hochschild, 1983/2003).

Another problematic aspect is that affective labor is framed by big data enthusiasts as something that occurs without the mediation of technology, when doctors can take their eyes away from computers and scans, and look instead at the patient. The findings presented here have shown, however, that digital technologies are an integral part of certain affective practices, shaping how people perform affective labor, and who the performers and recipients of affective labor can be. Studying affective labor online is important also because of the growing amount of value that is nowadays generated from the cognition, communication, affect, and the immaterial actions of online "prosumers" (Berardi, 2009; Hardt & Negri, 2004) and because scholars are divided about the role of such labor in digital media economics. Thus, many have criticized users' engagement with digital technologies as a form of free labor (Lupton, 2014; Mitchell & Waldby, 2010; Terranova, 2000; Waldby & Cooper, 2008), particularly since people are typically required to give up ownership over their data and any claims over potential profits that can be made from them. The findings presented in this book provide, however, a more nuanced perspective, as they show that online contributors perform affective labor in order to assist others, but they also benefit in various ways from these efforts, either because such practices contribute to their well-being or because they receive similar assistance from others, when they need it.

This book also showed that norms and values play an important role in the performance of expertise, not as sources of bias that need to be overcome, but as factors that motivate people to contribute in specific ways to knowledge production. Thus, Chap. 4 highlighted the role personal values and preferences play in how people assess treatment effectiveness and the therapeutic improvements or new treatments that they seek to contribute to, by sharing their personal experiences and insights. Whereas currently dominant neoliberal imperatives encourage individuals to assume responsibility for their health, the findings in Chap. 6 showed that lay expertise is importantly tied to the value of solidarity. These insights are aligned with the work of several philosophers of expertise (Goldman, 2018; Quast, 2018), who have highlighted the moral dimension of expertise. These authors have argued that people endowed with expertise are expected to behave responsibly, reflexively, and virtuously, and to assist others to the best of their abilities. While solidarity is largely neglected from such considerations, the findings presented in Chap. 6 suggest that it is a value that is worth paying more attention to in relation to expertise. By revealing the importance of affective labor for epistemic practices, this book helps expand the category of behaviors people endowed with expertise engage in and need to be aware of.

The findings of this book which highlighted the importance of communities for knowledge production are also important, as we currently "live in an environment in which datafied individualization of health responsibility appears like an inevitability" (McFall, 2019: 61). From this point of view, the Internet could be seen to finally live up to some of the visions it generated in its early days, when many expected it to lead to the development of virtual communities, as people with the same diagnosis could thus easily come together and talk about matters of interest, regardless of where they lived (Eysenbach, 2005; Hardey, 1999). By showing that people diagnosed with bipolar disorder perform expertise online, this book contributed to a growing body of literature (McFall, 2019; Prainsack & Buyx, 2017; Sharon, 2017; Van Hoyweghen & Rebert, 2012) that seeks to highlight the importance of this value in (mental) healthcare practices.

The conceptualization of expertise that I put forward highlights the complexity and diversity which characterize the production of knowledge in the digital age and the dynamic ways in which authority and influence can be (re)distributed among relevant stakeholders. This is important because in many situations a priori agreements about the identity of the "experts" or of the stakeholders involved in the development of expertise no longer hold, the relevance and impact of their input differ depending on the problem they are called to solve, and their role may change as new tools or practices are introduced (Waardenburg et al., 2018). From this point of view, the findings presented here constitute a contribution to the growing body of expertise studies, which emphasize the fact that nowadays individuals or groups socialized within different epistemic cultures have to intensely negotiate the relevance of their insights and the reach of their influence (Holst & Molander, 2018). By focusing on the knowledge with which different stakeholders are endowed, the new approach I put forward also highlights the importance not only of combining different types of theoretical knowledge, but of bringing together scientific insights with relevant local factors that only specific stakeholders may have knowledge of. This new conceptualization of expertise is thus in line with arguments recently provided by Barrotta and Montuschi (2018: 395), who state that "local knowledge coming from 'other sources' is often necessary to fill the gap between experts' knowledge and correct judgement calls." Another merit of this approach to expertise is that it draws attention to the importance of the ecosystem within which relevant stakeholders are based, as even sound recommendations may be thwarted or lead to less desirable effects depending on the available infrastructures, policies, legal provisions, and dominant political climate.

Through the findings presented, this book is therefore a contribution to the work of STS scholars who have cautioned against the hype surrounding digital technologies and their epistemic potential (Neff, 2013) and have argued, instead, that certain typically human capabilities continue to be very much needed in processes of knowledge production. These findings are thus important reminders of the value of nuanced perspectives, developed through rich, detailed studies, for a better understanding of the different functions and roles that people and digital technologies fulfill in processes of knowledge production. Whereas considering the online knowledge thus generated as mainly the merit of the technologies used would be a serious mistake, neglecting the active ways in which the latter do shape the content produced would be a danger that STS scholars have repeatedly warned against (Swierstra, 2016; Wyatt et al., 2016).

This book showed that different stakeholders performed expertise about bipolar disorder in different ways, depending on their skills and resources, on the ways in which they (could) chose to react to broader social transformations, and on the values that underpinned their engagements. The ways in which science and knowledge production are currently structured and organized increasingly require experts to make bold claims and to issue clear, unwavering recommendations about the problems they are called to solve. The varied and numerous accounts, doubts, and uncertainties expressed by the people diagnosed with bipolar disorder studied here constitute important reminders, however, that modesty, diversity of opinions, and constructive criticism are essential elements in the development of sound knowledge. By cultivating and enhancing the Internet's potential toward inclusive participation and (self)reflection, inquiries about the meaning and relevance of expertise will continue to generate enthusiasm, excitement, and heated debates. Many more exhilarating questions are thankfully opening up.

References

Barrotta, P., & Montuschi, E. (2018). Expertise, Relevance and Types of Knowledge. *Social Epistemology, 32*(6), 387–396.

Berardi, F. (2009). *The Soul at Work: From Alienation to Autonomy*. Semiotext (e).

Collins, H. (2018). *Artifictional Intelligence: Against Humanity's Surrender to Computers*. Polity Press. E-book.

Drucker, J. (2010). Graphesis. *Paj: The Journal of the Initiative for Digital Humanities, Media, and Culture, 2*(1), 1–50.

Engel, N., & Van Lente, H. (2014). Organizing Innovation and Control Practices: The Case of Public-Private Mix in Tuberculosis Control in India. *Sociology of Health and Illness, 36*(6), 917–931.

Eysenbach, G. (2005). Patient-to-Patient Communication: Support Groups and Virtual Communities. In D. Lewis, G. Eysenbach, R. Kukafka, P. Stavri, H. Jimison, & W. Slack (Eds.), *Consumer Health Informatics: Informing Consumers and Improving Health Care* (pp. 97–106). Springer.

Goldman, A. (2018). Expertise. *Topoi. An International Review of Philosophy, 37*(1), 3–10.

Hardey, M. (1999). Doctor in the House: The Internet as A Source of Lay Health Knowledge and the Challenge to Expertise. *Sociology of Healthy & Illness, 21*, 820–835.

Hardt, M., & Negri, A. (2004). *Multitude. War and Democracy in the Age of Empire*. The Penguin Press.

Hochschild A (2003/1983). *The Managed Heart. Commercialization of Human Feeling*. University of California Press.

Holst, C., & Molander, A. (2018). Asymmetry, Disagreement and Biases: Epistemic Worries about Expertise. *Social Epistemology, 32*(6), 358–371.

Van Hoyweghen, I., & Rebert, L. (2012). Your Genes in Insurance: From Generic Discrimination to Genomic Solidarity. *Personalized Medicine, 9*(8), 871–877.

Lupton, D. (2014). The Commodification of Patient Opinion: The Digital Patient Experience Economy in the Age of Big Data. *Sociology of Health & Illness, 36*(6), 856–869.

Mayer-Schönberger, V., & Cukier, K. (2013). *Big Data. A Revolution That Will Transform How We Live, Work and Think*. Houghton Mifflin Harcourt. E-book.

McFall, L. (2019). Personalizing Solidarity? The Role of Self-Tracking in Health Insurance Pricing. *Economy and Society, 48*(1), 52–76.

Mitchell, R., & Waldby, C. (2010). National Biobanks: Clinical Labor, Risk Production, and the Creation of Biovalue. *Science, Technology & Human Values, 35*(3), 330–355.

Neff, G. (2013). Why Big Data Won't Cure Us. *Big Data, 1*, 117–123. PMID:25161827.

Prainsack, B., & Buyx, A. (2017). *Solidarity in Biomedicine and Beyond*. Cambridge University Press.

Quast, C. (2018). Towards a Balanced Account of Expertise. *Social Epistemology, 32*(6), 397–419.

Sharon, T. (2017). Self-tracking for Health and the Quantified Self: Re-articulating Autonomy, Solidarity and Authenticity in an Age of Personalized Healthcare. *Philosophy & Technology, 30*(1), 93–121.

Swierstra, T. (2016). Introduction to the Ethics of New and Emerging Science and Technology. In R. Nakatsu, M. Rauterberg, & P. Ciancarini (Eds.),

Handbook of Digital Games and Entertainment Technologies (pp. 1271–1295). Springer.

Terranova, T. (2000). Free Labor: Producing Culture for the Digital Economy. *Social Text 63, 18*(2), 33–58.

Topol, E. (2019). *Deep Medicine. How Artificial Intelligence Can Make Healthcare Human Again.* Basic Books. E-book.

Waardenburg, L., Sergeeva, A., & Huysman, M. (2018). Hotspots and Blindspots: A Case of Predictive Policing in Practice. In U. Schultze, M. Mähring, L. Riemer, C. Østerlund, & M. Aanestad (Eds.), *IFIP Advances in Information and Communication Technology (543)* (pp. 96–109). Springer.

Waldby, C., & Cooper, M. (2008). The Biopolitics of Reproduction. *Australian Feminist Studies, 23*(55), 57–73.

Wyatt, S., Harris, A., & Kelly, S. (2016). Controversy Goes Online: Schizophrenia Genetics on Wikipedia. *Science & Technology Studies, 29*(1), 13–29.

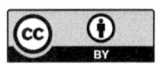

Index[1]

---

[1] Note: Page numbers followed by 'n' refer to notes.

© The Author(s) 2023   **245**
C. Egher, *Digital Healthcare and Expertise*, Health, Technology and Society,
https://doi.org/10.1007/978-981-16-9178-2